Pathology of Opportunistic Infections

Ramesh K. Gupta • Pallav Gupta
Editors

Pathology of Opportunistic Infections

An Illustrative Atlas

Springer

Editors
Ramesh K. Gupta
Department of Pathology
Sanjay Gandhi Postgraduate
Institute of Medical Sciences
Lucknow
India

Pallav Gupta
Department of Histopathology
Sir Ganga Ram Hospital
New Delhi
India

ISBN 978-981-10-1668-4 ISBN 978-981-10-1669-1 (eBook)
DOI 10.1007/978-981-10-1669-1

Library of Congress Control Number: 2016956857

Printed on acid-free paper

This Springer imprint is published by Springer Nature
The registered company is Springer Science+Business Media Singapore Pte Ltd.

To our patients and students

Foreword

It is a matter of pleasure for me to write this foreword for "Pathology of Opportunistic Infections: An Illustrative Atlas" authored by Prof. R. K. Gupta and Dr. Pallav Gupta. Professor Gupta is one of the pioneers in renal and transplant pathology in India. He has special interest in the pathology of opportunistic infections. His earlier book *Pathology of Opportunistic Infections in Tropics* is a testimony to his expertise and interest in this challenging field.

Over the past few decades, the science and practice of organ transplantation has advanced, providing optimal renal replacement therapy for patients with end-stage organ failure. Efforts are being made to improve the quality of life and prolong survival of transplant recipients throughout the world. However, in spite of prophylaxis for various transplant-associated infections, these immunocompromised patients are prone to acquire a variety of opportunistic infections, resulting in significant morbidity and mortality in individuals with otherwise well-functioning grafts. Clinical suspicion and early diagnosis of such infections are essential for prompt management of these cases. However, at times such infections remain underdiagnosed because of lack of awareness about the morphological features of such pathogens on cytopathological and/or histopathological examination.

The authors, applying their experience and expertise in the field, have included in this publication a large number of illustrative microphotographs of various opportunistic pathogens in different tissues and organs under diverse immunosuppressed states, supplementing succinct descriptions of pathological findings. This "Pathology of Opportunistic Infections: An Illustrative Atlas" should benefit transplant pathologists, microbiologists, immunologists, transplant physicians, and postgraduates, enabling prompt identification of opportunistic pathogens in tissues on cytopathological and/or histopathological examination.

Lorraine C. Racusen, MD
Department of Pathology
School of Medicine, The Johns Hopkins University,
Baltimore, MA, USA

Preface

The challenges posed by the opportunistic pathogens are enormous. Early clinical suspicion, prompt morphological identification, and timely management are essential to prevent high morbidity and mortality associated with these infections. These pathogens are often not identified because of the ignorance about their morphological appearances on histopathology and/or cytological evaluation. Although sufficient text is available on microbiological, serological, and molecular diagnosis of these infections, a comprehensive and updated illustrative presentation on the tissue identification of such infections is much needed, and the present illustrative atlas is aimed to fill this lacuna.

The authors having worked at a tertiary care medical center performing a large number of organ transplants in India encountered scores of opportunistic infections during histopathological and cytological evaluation of various specimens obtained from immunocompromised patients, which formed the basis of this illustrative atlas. This publication is entirely devoted to the morphological identification of opportunistic pathogens in various tissue specimens subjected to histopathological and/ or cytological evaluation in diverse clinical settings.

The atlas has a clearly organized layout with separate chapters dealing with opportunistic bacterial, viral, fungal, and parasitic infections along with a note on multiple opportunistic infections encountered in immunocompromised patients. Adequate references have also been provided in each chapter. The atlas includes more than 250 representative high-quality color microphotographs along with relevant clinical history of each case for easy identification by the readers. An appendix on the techniques and interpretation of commonly performed histochemical stains useful in the identification of these infections for the practicing pathologists has also been incorporated.

We hope that this illustrative and informative atlas on morphological identification of various opportunistic pathogens encountered in tissue specimen obtained from different lesions under diverse clinical settings as seen on histopathological and cytological examination shall be useful to a broad group of medical fraternity including transplant pathologists, microbiologists, physicians, nephrologists, immunologists, oncologists, transplant surgeons, and others as well.

Your suggestions and comments are most welcome.

Lucknow, India — Ramesh K. Gupta
New Delhi, India — Pallav Gupta

Acknowledgments

Readers of the earlier book entitled *Pathology of Opportunistic Infections in Tropics*, while expressing interest in this publication, suggested that to facilitate the morphological identification of various opportunistic infections in different tissues and organs under diverse clinical settings on histopathological and/or cytopathological examination, high-quality microphotographs of the morphological details of different opportunistic pathogens should be provided. It encouraged us to bring out this illustrative atlas on the subject. We are indeed grateful to the readers for their feedback and valuable suggestions.

Majority of the cases included in this atlas are from our own experience, while others have been contributed by friends and colleagues from other institutes.

We gratefully acknowledge the contribution of some of the interesting cases by Prof. Kusum Joshi, head of the Department of Histopathology, Postgraduate Institute of Medical Education and Research, Chandigarh; Prof. Harsh Mohan, head of the Department of Pathology, Government Medical College, Chandigarh; Prof. S. K. Shankar, professor emeritus and director of the Human Brain Bank, National Institute of Mental Health and Neurosciences, Bangalore; Prof. K. N. Prasad, Department of Microbiology, and Prof. Narendra Krishnani, Prof. Manoj Jain, and Prof Vinita Agrawal, Department of Pathology, Sanjay Gandhi Postgraduate Institute of Medical Sciences, Lucknow; Dr. Silista Radha and Dr. Tameem Afroz, consultant pathologists, Aware Global Hospital, Hyderabad; Dr. Anjali Amrapurkar, associate professor, Department of Pathology, Nair Hospital, Mumbai; and Dr. Vipul Srivastava, consultant microbiologist, and Dr. Shalini Bhalla, consultant pathologist, Sahara Hospital, Lucknow. We are also grateful to M/S Medknow, the publishers of "Neurology India" and M/S Jaypee Brothers Medical Publishers (P) Ltd, New Delhi, the publishers of earlier book "Pathology of Opportunistic Infections in Tropics" for permitting to use some of the contents published earlier by them. We are also grateful to all our colleagues and friends for extending all possible support in the compilation of this atlas. We are grateful to Prof. Lorraine C. Racusen, the Johns Hopkins University School of Medicine, Baltimore, Maryland, USA, for writing the foreword of this book.

We are thankful to the publishers Springer Science+Business Media Singapore Pte Ltd., Singapore, for publishing and making this atlas presentable.

Contents

About the Author

R.K. Gupta Professor Gupta is a medical graduate (MBBS) and postgraduate MD (Path. & Bact.) from King George's Medical College, Lucknow. He was awarded several prizes and honors both during his undergraduate and postgraduate medical career. After having served in various academic positions such as assistant professor, associate professor, and professor for about 20 years in UP State Government Medical Colleges, in the year 1992, he joined as professor and head of the Department of Pathology at the Sanjay Gandhi Postgraduate Institute of Medical Sciences, Lucknow. At this upcoming medical institute, he developed the Department of Pathology to its best and initiated MD (pathology) postgraduate course and established specialty pathology training and postdoctorate certificate course in renal pathology. At Sanjay Gandhi PGI, he made tremendous academic and administrative contributions and had also been the dean and director of the institute.

Professor Gupta has keen interest in research. Renal pathology, transplant pathology, cardiac pathology, and pathology of opportunistic infections have been some of the specialized areas of his academic activities. He has completed more than 20 research projects funded by international, national, and regional scientific bodies and has contributed more than 140 original research articles in various national and international journals of high repute. He has several book references and book chapters to his credit and has published five manuals and proceedings and a book on *Pathology of Opportunistic Infections in Tropics*.

Professor Gupta has more than 45 years of professional and academic experience to his credit. During this period, he had been the guide and mentor to more than 50 postgraduates in the speciality of pathology and allied sciences. He is recognized as an academician of high repute by the peers and has been invited to present several prestigious orations and guest lectures at various national and international scientific meets. For his academic contributions, he has been conferred with several honors and awards including prestigious Fellowship of National Academy of Medical Sciences (India). Professor Gupta has most successfully organized several national and international scientific meets including the APCON Gold the golden jubilee IAPM National Conference, 3rd International CME on Surgical Pathology, and 1st International CME on Renal Pathology. He has held high offices of vice-president and president of the Indian Association of Pathologists and Microbiologists and several other national academic bodies. In 2005, he formed the Indian Society of Renal and Transplant Pathology, of which he had been the founding president. He had been on the editorial board of some of the prestigious medical journals and a reviewer to various scientific and academic bodies.

Pallav Gupta Dr. Pallav Gupta, a postgraduate in pathology, has obtained specialized training and a postdoctorate certificate in the field of renal and transplant pathology. He is a diagnostic histopathologist of repute, and special areas of his academic interest include renal and transplant pathology. He is presently working as a consultant pathologist and renal pathologist at Sir Ganga Ram Hospital, New Delhi. He is DNB thesis guide for postgraduates in pathology and has authored more than 25 publications in peer-reviewed national and international journals. In recognition of his academic achievements, he has been awarded MAMS by the National Academy of Medical Sciences (NAMS), New Delhi, India. He is also an executive member of the Indian Society of Renal and Transplant Pathology besides being a life member of several national and international academic bodies. He is a reviewer of several international journals.

Introduction to Opportunistic Infections

1

During the last few decades, certain clinical and therapeutic developments, such as the HIV/AIDS pandemic, advances in organ transplantation, cancer chemoradiotherapy, prolonged use of steroids, and other immunosuppressants for various autoimmune diseases while prolonging patient survival, have also created major aberrations in host defense mechanisms, thereby increasing the vulnerability of these patients to a variety of opportunistic infections.

Further, the increasing use of certain therapeutic procedures and interventions like prolonged use of central lines, IV canulae, indwelling catheters, shunts, postoperative states, peritoneal and hemodialysis, postinfective states, and many other debilitating disease states and other clinical conditions such as diabetes mellitus, major organ compromises like chronic kidney diseases (CKD), chronic liver diseases (CLD), and chronic lung diseases also lead to altered immune responses, therefore, predisposing the patients to infections with opportunistic pathogens. The patients at extremes of age such as neonates and infants due to immature immune system and the elderly due to abrasions in immune responses are also at risk of contracting various opportunistic infections. Therefore, due to unusual clinical presentation and lack of early detection, often these infections, and not the primary illness, significantly contribute to the associated morbidity and mortality in such patients.

Immunocompromised states lead to impairment of natural/specific immunity causing increased risk to infections by a variety of microorganisms, which can broadly be classified into three categories.

1. "*True pathogens*" possess virulence to overcome natural host resistance.
2. "*Sometime pathogens*" are normal colonizers of mucocutaneous surfaces and cause clinical disease only when introduced into the tissues following a breach in the integrity of the mucocutaneous barrier; once introduced, these organisms possess sufficient virulence to cause lethal infections.
3. "*Nonpathogens*" are the organisms generally susceptible to natural body resistance supplemented by specific immunity. However, they can cause disease in individuals with impaired immunity.

The term opportunistic infection(s) is used either for invasive infection(s) due to "nonpathogens" (*Pneumocystis carinii*, *Aspergillus fumigatus*, etc.) or to denote infection(s) due to "true" or "sometime pathogens" which are of a type or severity rarely encountered in an immunocompetent host. Hepatosplenic candidiasis in leukemic patients and disseminated herpes infection or recurrent salmonellosis in AIDS are some examples of such infections.

R.K. Gupta, P. Gupta (eds.), *Pathology of Opportunistic Infections*,
DOI 10.1007/978-981-10-1669-1_1

Factors Influencing Host Defense Mechanisms

Various factors may be responsible for lowering of natural/specific host resistance. The extremes of age predispose to opportunistic infections by virtue of immature immune system in neonates and infants and impaired repair mechanisms in elderly. Disease states like diabetes mellitus, chronic liver disease, chronic renal failure, malignancies, malnutrition, and also as yet undetermined genetic factors also predispose to opportunistic infections. Major aberrations of innate/acquired immunity in common clinical practice are due to:

1. *Granulocytopenia*: As the granulocyte count falls below 500/µl, the frequency of infections tend to increase. Infection is also more likely to occur with rapidly falling counts than in the setting of stable granulocytopenia as observed in conditions like aplastic anemia or benign idiopathic neutropenia. Granulocytopenia is frequently observed after the administration of chemotherapy and/or radiations. Organ transplant recipients may also experience myelosuppression while receiving cyclophosphamide or azathioprine. Defects in immune functions are further enhanced by the addition of steroids. In the presence of granulocytopenia, normal colonizers of the mucosa invade and establish infection. *E. coli*, *K. pneumoniae*, and *P. aeruginosa* are the most common Gram-negative pathogens encountered in granulocytopenic patients, while *S. aureus* and coagulase-negative staphylococci are important Gram-positive coccal pathogens. The use of broad-spectrum antibiotics further provides an opportunity for overgrowth by yeast and filamentous fungi, such as *Candida* species, *Torulopsis glabrata*, and *Aspergillus*.
2. *Cellular immune dysfunction*: Patients with lymphoma, HIV/AIDS, etc., have an inherent abnormality in cellular immune functions. Similar alterations may also develop as a result of drug reactions, radiation therapy, or immunosuppression associated with organ transplantation. Relatively few organisms cause infection in these settings, most being intracellular pathogens. Bacterial infections encountered in these patients include *Listeria monocytogenes*, *Salmonella*, typical and atypical *Mycobacteria*, and *Legionella pneumophila*. Viruses like varicella zoster, CMV, EBV, and respiratory syncytial virus (RSV) and fungi like, *Cryptococcus*, *Histoplasma*, and *Coccidioides* are also important pathogens in this group of patients. It is important to emphasize that in many patients, the illness is caused by reactivation of a latent or dormant infection. Infections by protozoan parasites such as *Toxoplasma gondii*, *Cryptosporidium,* and *Microspora* and helminths such as *Strongyloides stercoralis* are also not uncommon in these patients.
3. *Humoral immune dysfunction*: Patients with multiple myeloma and chronic lymphocytic leukemia are either hypogammaglobulinemic or produce abnormal paraproteins which do not have adequate opsonizing capabilities for encapsulated organisms like *Streptococcus pneumoniae* or *Haemophilus influenzae*.
4. *Obstruction of natural body passages*: Partial or complete obstruction of natural body orifices or passages leads to infection because of stasis of body fluids and overgrowth of native colonizing microorganisms. Examples include post-obstruction pneumonias in patients with lung tumors, ascending cholangitis secondary to biliary obstruction, and urinary tract infections caused by obstructing prostatic, rectal, ovarian, or cervical malignancies. Infections in these patients are almost exclusively bacterial with anaerobic organisms playing a significant role in the pathogenesis.
5. *Iatrogenic procedures*: Immunocompromised patients most often undergo a series of

medical and surgical interventions/procedures including catheterizations, venipunctures, marrow aspirations, and also blood and blood product transfusions or parenteral nutrition. These procedures may also predispose the immunocompromised patients to a variety of opportunistic infections.

Common Opportunistic Infections

Immunocompromised hosts invariably suffer with repeated opportunistic infections which at times may be multiple. Different bacterial, viral, fungal, and parasitic microbes contribute to majority of these infections (Table 1.1).

Table 1.1 Common opportunistic pathogens

Bacterial	Viral	Fungal	Parasitic
Salmonella	Herpes simplex	*Candida*	*Giardia lamblia*
Encapsulated bacteria	Herpes zoster	*Cryptococcus*	*Entamoeba*
Mycobacterium tuberculosis	CMV	*Pneumocystis carinii*	*Toxoplasma*
Mycobacterium avium complex	HVB	*Histoplasma*	*Leishmania*
Nocardia	HPV	Coccidioidomycosis	*Isospora*
		Aspergillus	*Cryptosporidium*
		Zygomycetes	Microsporidium
			Strongyloidosis

Prevalence of Opportunistic Infections

In various clinical subset of patients such as solid organ transplantation, HIV/AIDS, and granulocytopenia, depending upon the type and severity of immunosuppression, the prevalence and time of occurrence of various opportunistic infections differs widely in various reported series (Tables 1.2, 1.3 and 1.4).

Table 1.2 Time of occurrence of various opportunistic infections after solid organ transplantation

<1 month	1–6 months	>6 months
Bacteremias	CMV, EBV	Cryptococcosis
Candidiasis	Viral hepatitis	*Listeria monocytogenes*
	Nocardia	*Nocardia*
	Pneumocystis carinii	*Pneumocystis carinii*
	Aspergillosis	

Table 1.3 Prevalence of common fungal infections in patients of AIDS, solid organ transplantation, and granulocytopenia

	AIDS	Organ transplant	Granulocytopenia
Pneumocystis carinii	80 %	Infrequent	Infrequent
Mucocutaneous candidiasis	90 %	70 %	48 %
Systemic candidiasis	Rare	Rare	Rare
Systemic cryptococcosis	5–12 %	Rare	Rare
Histoplasmosis	2–5 %	Rare	Rare
Coccidioidomycosis	5 %	–	–
Aspergillosis	Infrequent	25 %	31 %

Table 1.4 Prevalence of common viral infections in solid organ and bone marrow transplant recipients

Viral infection	Solid organ transplant	Bone marrow transplant	
CMV	50–60 %	2–7 %	Autologous
		10–40 %	Allogenic
EBV	5 %	<1 %	
H. zoster	3 %	25 %	Autologous
		40 %	Allogenic
H. simplex	40 %	–	
Papovavirus	30 %	–	
HPV	42 %	–	

2 Opportunistic Bacterial Infections

Bacterial organisms even of low virulence may cause local or disseminated infections in immunocompromised patients. In these patients the inflammatory response is impaired with masking of signs and symptoms. Various immunocompromised states leading to enhanced vulnerability to bacterial infections are:

1. *Defective cell-mediated immunity*: These patients are prone to infections with intracellular organisms, e.g., mycobacteria, nocardia, and salmonella.
2. *Defective humoral immunity*: These patients are prone to infections with encapsulated bacteria, e.g., *S. pneumoniae* and *H. influenzae*.
3. *Granulocytopenia*: These patients are prone to infections with Gram-negative bacilli, e.g., *E. coli*, *Klebsiella*, and *P. aeruginosa*.

Some of the bacterial infections elicit distinct morphological alterations and can be diagnosed on histopathological or cytopathological evaluation. However, majority of bacterial infections do not induce specific tissue reaction; therefore the "gold standard" for the diagnosis of these infections continues to be bacterial culture. The specimen for bacterial culture should be obtained prior to antibiotic therapy.

Mycobacterium Tuberculosis: Two species of mycobacteria, *M. tuberculosis* and *M. bovis*, cause tuberculosis in man. *M. tuberculosis* is usually transmitted through airborne droplets; however both *M. tuberculosis* and *M. bovis* may also be transmitted through contaminated milk. In primary infection the organisms cause localized pulmonary disease. In immunocompromised host, the primary infection may progress to cavitation, pneumonia, or disseminated infection. A defective immune response leads to ill-formed granulomas with large areas of necrosis harboring abundant tubercle bacilli. Characteristic clinical manifestations are often occult; tuberculin test is not useful in these patients; however on Ziehl-Neelsen staining, sputum samples often reveal heavy positivity for acid-fast bacilli. Besides culture, PCR helps in rapid identification.

R.K. Gupta, P. Gupta (eds.), *Pathology of Opportunistic Infections*,
DOI 10.1007/978-981-10-1669-1_2

Besides *M. tuberculosis*, the immunocompromised individuals are also susceptible to infection with certain opportunistic mycobacteria. Two closely related species of mycobacteria, *M. avium* and *M. intracellulare*, together form *Mycobacterium avium complex (MAC)*. MAC complex causes lymphadenitis, skin lesions, lung involvement, and disseminated disease in immunocompromised host. Profound diarrhea may be seen in patients with gastrointestinal involvement. MAC infection is usually resistant to most of the antimycobacterial agents.

In these patients, the lesions may not show characteristic well-formed epithelioid granulomas on histological or cytopathological evaluation; rather ill-formed epithelioid granulomas against necrotic background may be seen. However, these lesions are often heavily positive for acid-fast bacilli on Ziehl-Neelsen stain.

FNA-Tubercular Lymphadenitis in a Renal Allograft Recipient

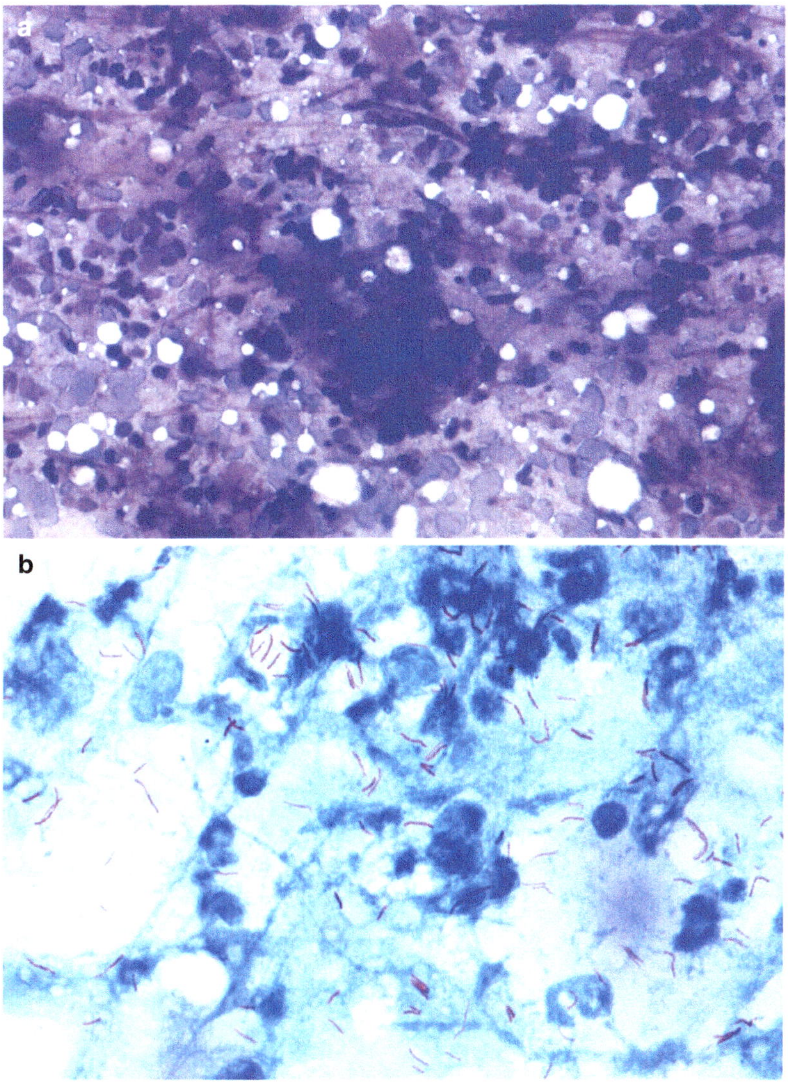

Fig. 2.1 (**a**, **b**) A 30-year-old male patient receiving live-related renal allograft 10 years back otherwise having stable renal function presented with mild pain in the abdomen and low-grade fever for the past 1 year. USG abdomen revealed enlargement of para-aortic lymph nodes; guided FNA showed degenerate leukocytes intermixed with few histiocytes, ill-defined collections of epithelioid cells, and foamy macrophages against necrotic background (**a** MGG ×400). Ziehl-Neelsen stain showed plenty of acid-fast bacilli (**b** ZN stain ×1000) (Contributor – Prof. Manoj Jain, Department of Pathology, Sanjay Gandhi Postgraduate Institute of Medical Sciences, Lucknow, India)

Tubercular Lymphadenitis in a Renal Allograft Recipient

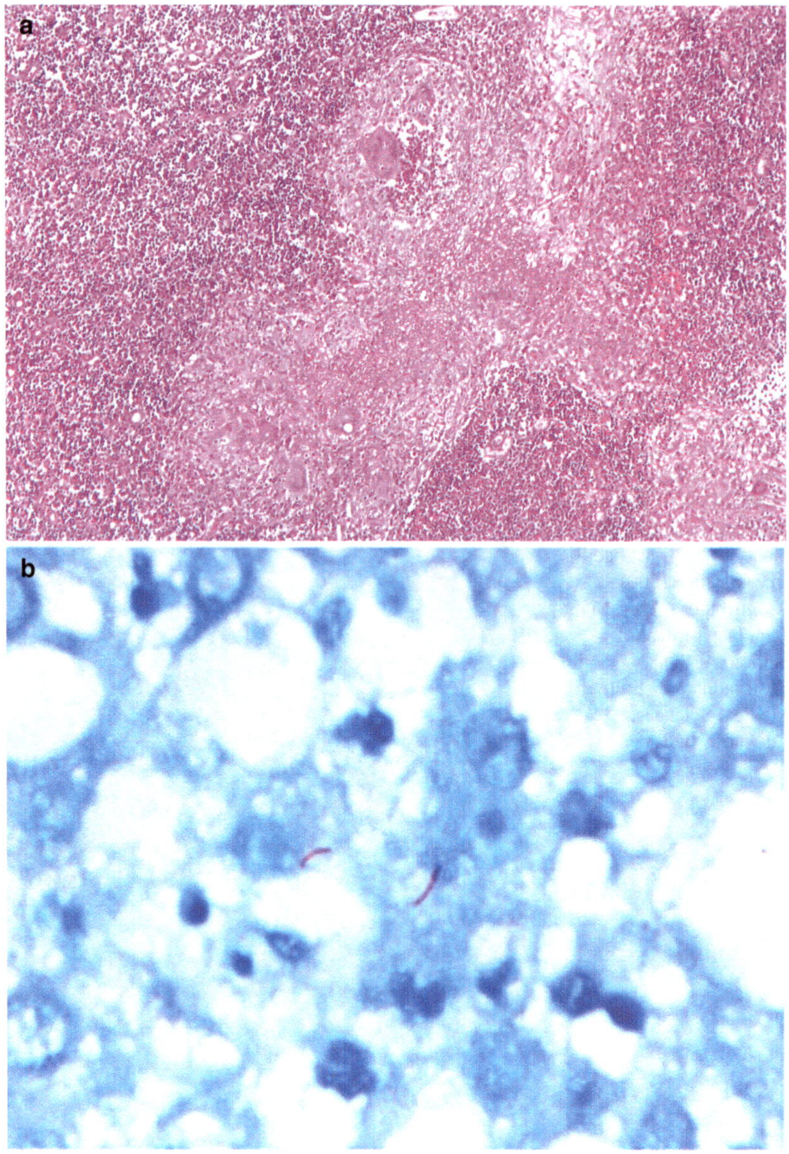

Fig. 2.2 (**a**, **b**) A 35-year-old male patient who received live-related renal allograft 15 months back and was being maintained on triple-drug immunosuppression presented with low-grade fever and left cervical lymphadenopathy for 2 months. The lymph node biopsy showed well-formed multiple coalescing epithelioid granulomas along with multiple Langhans giant cells and central caseation (**a** HE ×100). Ziehl-Neelsen stain showed few acid-fast bacilli at the periphery of necrotic areas (**b** ZN ×1000). Histological diagnosis of tubercular lymphadenitis was offered

Tubercular Lymphadenitis in a HIV-Positive Patient

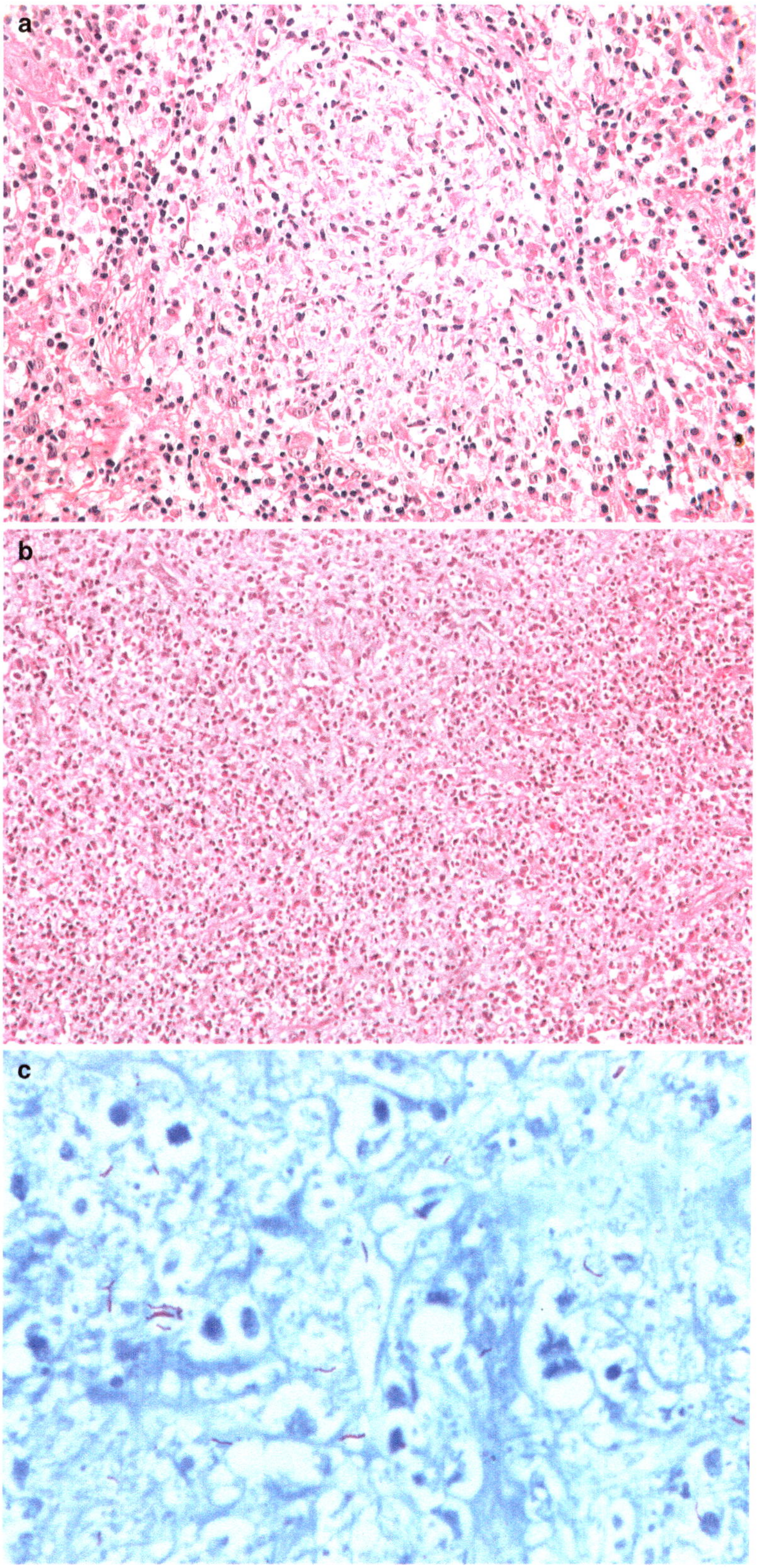

Fig. 2.3 (**a**–**c**) A 36-year-old HIV-positive male patient presented with fever associated with evening rise of temperature since 2 months with h/o weight loss and loss of appetite. On examination he was found to have bilateral cervical and axillary lymphadenopathy. There was no hepatosplenomegaly. The X-ray chest (PA) was WNL. Routine hematological workup revealed Hb content of 10.1 g/dl, total WBC count 9200/cu mm with neutrophils 40, lymphocytes 52, eosinophils 3, and monocytes 5 %, respectively. ESR was 58 mm. CD4 count was 85/cu mm. Excisional axillary lymph node biopsy showed ill-defined epithelioid granulomas against necrotic background along with inflammatory infiltrate (**a**, **b** HE ×200). Ziehl-Neelsen stain showed fair number of acid-fast bacilli in the necrotic areas (**c** ZN ×1000)

FNA-Tubercular Lymphadenitis in a HIV-Positive Patient

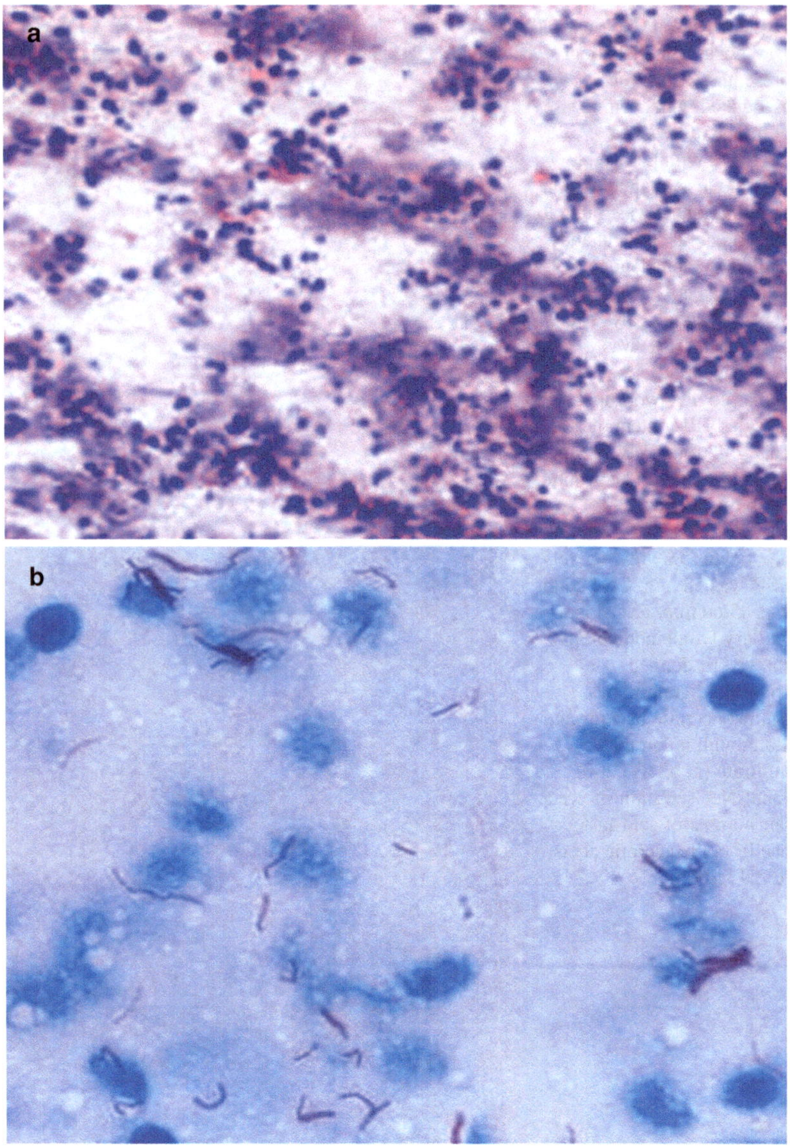

Fig. 2.4 (**a**, **b**) A 28-year-old male taxi driver by profession presented with PUO, weight loss, generalized weakness, and persistent generalized lymphadenopathy for 3 months. FNAC from the cervical lymph node revealed mixed inflammatory infiltrate against a necrotic background (**a** MGG ×200). Ziehl-Neelsen stain revealed the presence of large number of acid-fast bacilli (**b** ZN ×1000). Subsequent investigations revealed that the patient was HIV positive with CD4 counts of 120/cu mm

Tuberculosis Liver in an Immunocompromised Patient

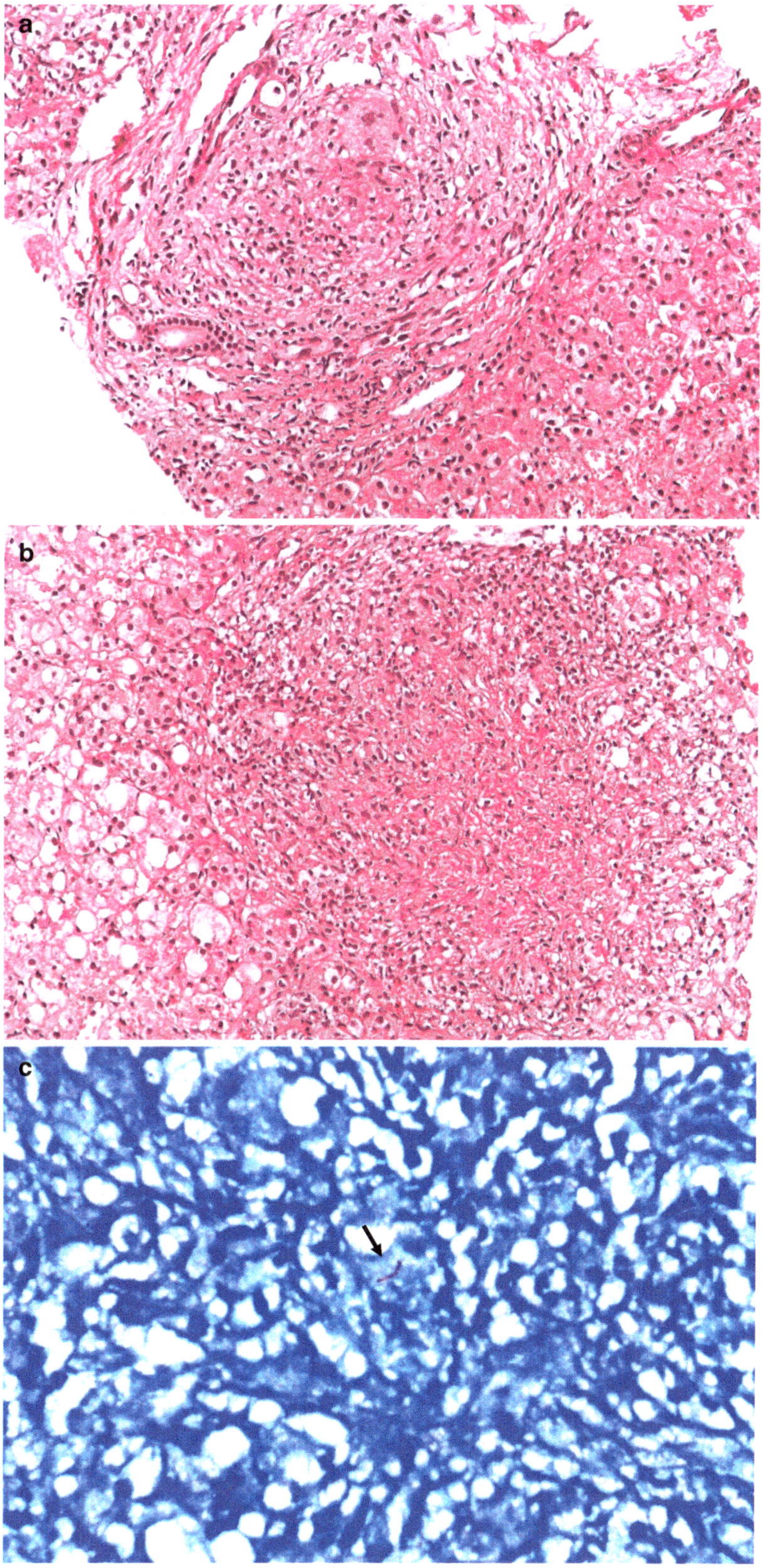

Fig. 2.5 (**a–c**) A 41-year-old female patient, known case of SLE on long term prednisolone, presented with fever, weight loss (6 kg), and loss of appetite since 2 months. Laboratory workup revealed Hb 10.5 g/dl, TLC 9200/mm with P52 L47 E1 M2%, respectively. Platelet count was 160,000/cu mm. Liver function tests were mildly deranged with S. bilirubin 2.1 mg/dl, SGOT 84 U/L, and SGPT 90 U/L. USG abdomen showed multiple hypoechoic lesions in both lobes of the liver and spleen with abdominal lymphadenopathy. Ultrasound-guided Tru-Cut liver biopsy showed multiple noncaseating epithelioid granulomas in periportal areas (**a** HE ×200) as well as in other parts of the liver parenchyma (**b** HE ×200); Ziehl-Neelsen stain revealed occasional acid-fast bacilli (**c** ZN ×1000) (*arrow*)

Tubercular Interstitial Nephritis in Renal Allograft

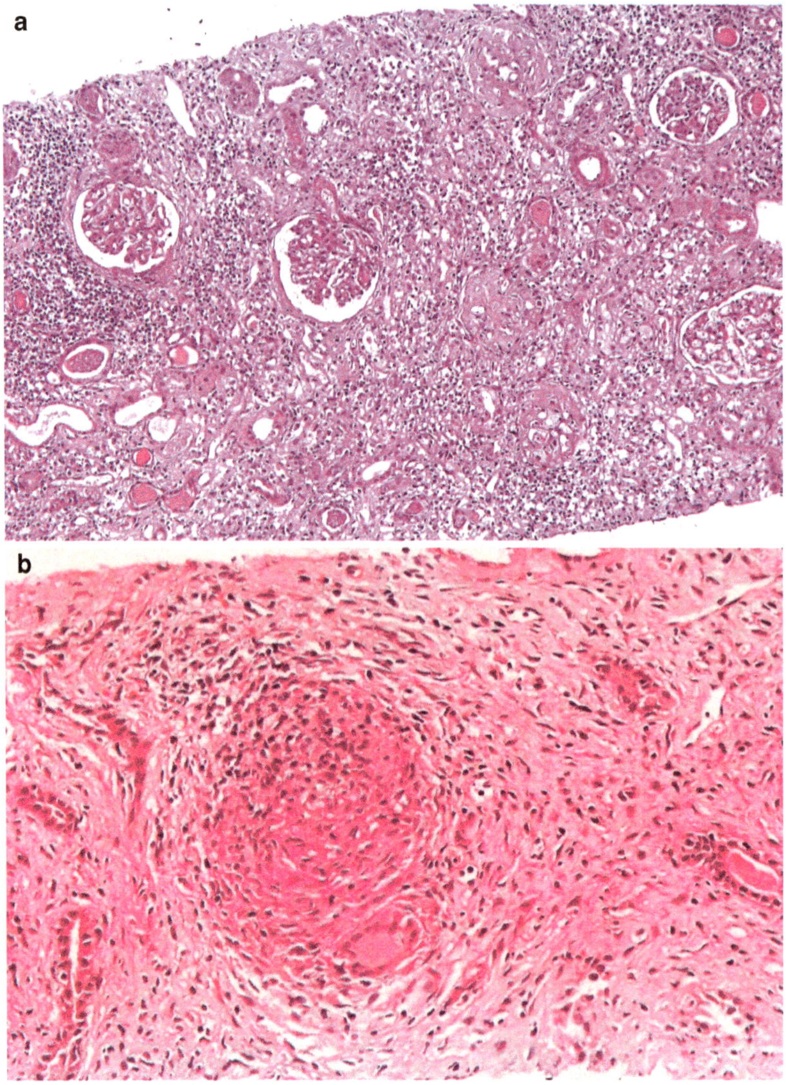

Fig. 2.6 (**a**, **b**) A 34-year-old female patient receiving live-related ABO compatible renal allograft, about 2 years post-Tx, presented with low-grade intermittent fever with evening rise of temperature without chills and rigors for 15 days; she also had mild cough with scanty mucoid expectoration accompanied with constitutional symptoms such as fatigue, weakness, and anorexia; there was no dyspnea, hemoptysis, or palpitation. X-ray chest (PA) and USG and Doppler of the graft kidney were WNL. Laboratory workup revealed hemoglobin content of 11.9 g/dl, TLC was 9200/cu mm with 46 % lymphocytes. Platelets were 1.57 L/cu mm; ESR was 66 mm at first hour. Serum creatinine was 2.03 mg/dl. Total serum protein was 6 g/dl with albumin being 2.8 g/dl. LFT was WNL. Urine P/C ratio was 1.98. Urine examination showed mild albuminuria (1+) with 5–10 wbc/phf. Urine culture was sterile. Serology for HBsAg, HCV, and HIV 1 and 2, dengue, malaria, and typhoid was negative. Serum tacrolimus C0 level was 101 pg, and C2 level was 403 pg/ml. Sputum smears did not show any AFB or fungal elements; sputum culture did not grow any organisms. At this stage CT chest was undertaken which revealed multiple millimeter size ill-defined diffusely scattered lesions in bilateral lung parenchyma and mildly enlarged left para-aortic lymph nodes; QuantiFERON gold test was positive. Renal allograft biopsy revealed tubulointerstitial nephritis with the presence of compact noncaseating epithelioid cell granulomas along with Langhans giant cells; however any AFB could not be demonstrated on ZN stain (**a** HE ×100, **b** HE ×400)

Nocardia: *Nocardia* are aerobic filamentous bacteria occurring as environmental saprophytes. The infection is acquired by inhalation of bacilli. Lung involvement commonly presents as pneumonia. Acute dissemination of the infection with multi-organ involvement occurs in immunocompromised patients.

Nocardial filaments are 1 μm wide with branching at right angles and appear basophilic in HE stained sections. Gram stain shows irregular beaded/granular appearance. The organism is partially acid fast and non-alcohol fast (Kinyoun, Fite-Faraco stains). The bacilli appear argyrophilic on GMS stain.

Nocardia Lung in a Renal Allograft Recipient

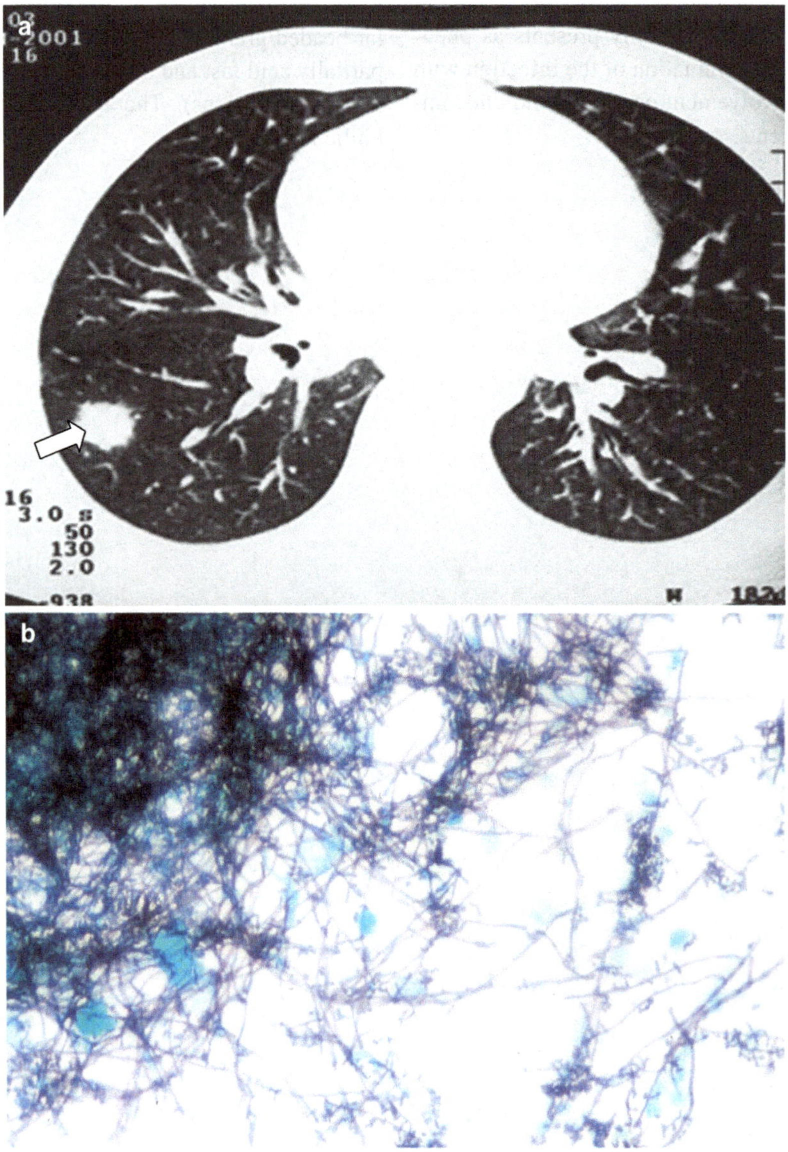

Fig. 2.7 (**a**, **b**) A 32-year-old male patient who received live-related renal allograft 6 years back was on triple-drug immunosuppression consisting of cyclosporine, azathioprine, and wysolone. He presented with generalized weakness, breathlessness, and right-sided chest pain for 2 months. CT chest revealed a solitary nodule in the right lower lobe (**a**). FNAC from the lesion showed filamentous branching organisms suggestive of *Nocardia* (**b** GSM ×400) (Contributors – S. Radha and Tameem Afroz, Aware Global Hospital, Hyderabad, India)

Nocardial Brain Abscess in a HIV-Positive Patient

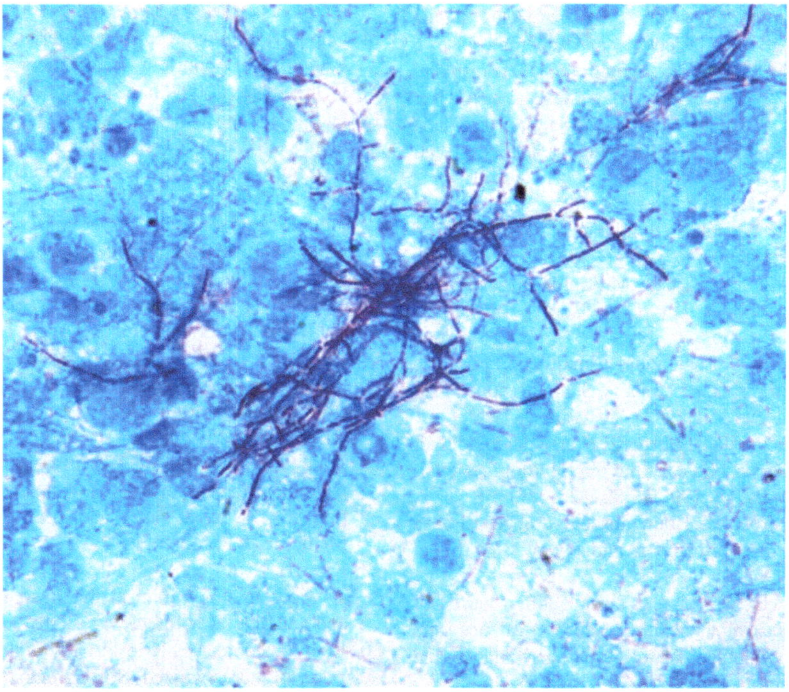

Fig. 2.8 A 40-year-old male patient presented with headache and seizures for 3 months and altered sensorium for 15 days. Radiological investigations revealed a frontoparietal ring-enhancing lesion. On surgery, the lesion was found to be an abscess which was drained. Examination of pus showed Gram-positive and acid-fast filamentous bacilli (Ziehl-Neelsen ×400). Culture on blood agar medium showed the growth of *Nocardia*. Further investigations revealed that the patient was HIV positive with CD4 counts of 36/cu mm (Contributor – Prof. K N Prasad, Department of Microbiology, Sanjay Gandhi Postgraduate Institute of Medical Sciences, Lucknow, India)

Further Reading

1. Agarwal DK, Mehta AK, Sharma AP, Sural S, Kumar A, Mehta B, Gupta A, Sharma RK, Gupta RK. Coinfection with leprosy and tuberculosis in a renal transplant recipient. Nephrol Dial Transplant. 2000;15:1720–1.
2. Beaman L, Beaman BL. Nocardia species: host parasite relationships. Clin Microbiol Rev. 1994; 7:213–64.
3. Bloom BR, Small PM. The evolving relation between humans and Mycobacterium tuberculosis. N Eng J Med. 1998;338:677–8.
4. Bradfard WZ, Daley CL. Multiple drug resistant tuberculosis. Infect Dis Clin North Am. 1998; 12:157–72.
5. Chow J, Yw VL. Legionella: a major opportunistic infection in transplant recipients. Semin Respir Infect. 1998;13:132–9.
6. Coker RJ, Bignarde G, Horner P, et al. Nocardia infection in AIDS: a clinical and microbiological challenge. J Clin Pathol. 1992;45:821–2.
7. Dee RR, Lorber B. Brain abscess due to Listeria monocytogenes: case report and review. Rev Infect Dis. 1986;8:968–77.
8. Dye C, Scheele S, Dolin P, et al. Global burden of tuberculosis: estimated incidence, prevalence and mortality by country. WHO global surveillance and monitoring project. JAMA. 1999;282:677–86.
9. Edelstein PH, Meyer RD. Legionella pneumonias. In: Pennington GE, editor. Respiratory infection: diagnosis and management. New York: Raven Press; 1994. p. 455–84.
10. Farina C, Borion P, Goglio A, et al. Human nocardiosis in northern Italy from 1982–1992. Northern Italy collaborative group on nocardiosis. Scand J Infect Dis. 1995;27:23–7.
11. Gaillard JL, Berche P, Frehel C, Govin E, Cossart P. Entry of L. Monocytogenes into cells is mediated by internalin, a repeat protein reminiscent of surface antigens from gram positive cocci. Cell. 1991;65:1127–41.
12. Grange JM. Actinomyces and nocardia. In: David G, Richard S, John P, editors. Medical microbiology – a guide to microbial infections: pathogenesis, immunity, laboratory diagnosis and control. 15th ed. New York: Churchill Livingstone; 1997. p. 222.
13. Gupta RK. Opportunistic infections in renal allograft recipients. Transplant Proc. 2007;39:731–3.
14. Gupta RK. Opportunistic bacterial infections. In: Pathology of opportunistic infections in tropics. New Delhi: Jaypee; 2007. p. 4.
15. Gupta P, Rana DS, Bhalla AK, Gupta A, Malik M, Gupta A, Bhargava V. Renal failure due to granulomatous interstitial nephritis in native and allograft renal biopsies: experience from a tertiary care hospital. Ren Fail. 2014;36(9):1468–70.
16. Heidrun R. Pathology of infectious diseases. In: Connor DH, Chandler FW, et al., editors. Mycobacterium avium complex (MAC) infection, vol. 1. Stamford: Appleton & Lange; 1997. p. 657.
17. Horsburgh Jr CR, Metchok BG, Mc Gowan JE, et al. Clinical implications of recovery of MAC from the stool or respiratory tract of HIV-infected individuals. AIDS. 1992;6:512–4.
18. Janaly K, Horowitz HW, Wormser GP. Nocardiosis in patients with human immunodeficiency virus infection: report of 2 cases and review of literature. Medicine (Baltimore). 1992;71:128–38.
19. Kim JH, Langston AA, Gallis HA. Miliary tuberculosis: epidemiology, clinical manifestations, diagnosis and outcome. Rev Infect Dis. 1990;12:583–90.
20. Kool JL, Fiore AE, Krioski CM, et al. More than 10 years of unrecognized Nosocomial transmission of legionnaires disease among transplant patients. Infect Control Hosp Epidemiol. 1998;9:898–904.
21. Kramer MR, Uttamchandani RB. The radiographic appearance of pulmonary nocardiosis associated with AIDS. Chest. 1990;98:382–5.
22. Muray EGD, Webb RE, Swann MBR. A disease of rabbits characterized by a large mononuclear leukocytosis, caused by a hitherto undescribed bacillus bacterium monocytogenes. J Pathol Bacterial. 1926;27:407–39.
23. Murray EGD. The story of Listeria. Trans Roy Sec Can. 1953;47:15–21.
24. Nieman RE, Lorber B. Listeriosis in adults: a changing pattern. Report of eight cases and review of literature. Rev Infect Dis. 1980;2:207–27.
25. Young LS. The garrod lecture. Mycobacterial disease in the 1990s. J Antimicrob Chemother. 1993;32:179–94.

3 Opportunistic Viral Infections

Viral infections most often represent reactivation of latent or subclinical infection in immunocompromised host. Both viral and host factors determine the susceptibility to infection. The susceptibility and severity of viral infections increases in conditions with inherited or acquired immunodeficiency, immunosuppressive drug therapy, or transplant recipients or in patients with compromised cellular immunity, e.g., AIDS.

The laboratory techniques utilized for the diagnosis of viral infections include direct visualization (cytology, histology, and electron microscopy), viral culture, detection of viral antigens (radioimmunoassay, enzyme immunoassay, and immunofluorescence), and serological detection of antibodies. Currently molecular techniques based on the detection of viral genome are being increasingly used for the diagnosis of viral infections.

Commonly encountered opportunistic viral pathogens are listed in Table 3.1.

Herpes Simplex Virus (HSV): Herpes simplex virus (HSV) includes two serotypes HSV 1 and HSV 2. HSV can involve any organ or mucocutaneous site. However, HSV 1 is usually said to affect upper half of the body causing oral lesions and HSV 2 the lower half, involving genital organs. Neonatal herpes simplex is caused by HSV 2 in 70 % and by HSV 1 in 30 % cases. The infection is acquired during vaginal delivery and can be prevented by cesarean section.

Immunocompromised patients show extensive lesions and frequently develop disseminated disease involving the esophagus, upper respiratory tract, lung, and liver. Other organs like the adrenals, pancreas, intestine, and bone marrow may also be involved.

Microscopic examination reveals that the epithelial cells lining the vesicular cutaneous and mucosal lesions show eosinophilic homogenous cytoplasm and nucleomegaly with viral inclusions. The inclusions are 3–8 μm, round to oval, amphophilic, and homogenous with ground glass appearance surrounded by a halo, and multinucleation may also be present.

Tzanck smear can be prepared for rapid preliminary diagnosis. Cytological specimen like vesicular fluid and scrapings from the base of the lesions stained with Giemsa, Papanicolaou, or toluidine blue may show characteristic giant cells and acantholytic balloon cells with intranuclear inclusions of herpes. In herpes pneumonia, bronchial biopsy and brushings may show characteristic viral inclusions in alveolar lining cells. Immunohistochemistry and fluorescent techniques with specific antibodies can be applied on paraffin-embedded tissue.

R.K. Gupta, P. Gupta (eds.), *Pathology of Opportunistic Infections*,
DOI 10.1007/978-981-10-1669-1_3

Table 3.1 Common opportunistic viral pathogens

Family	Subfamily	Example
DNA viruses		
ds DNA viruses		
Herpesviridae	*Alphaherpesvirinae*	
	Simplex virus	Human herpes virus 1 and 2 (HSV)
	Varicella virus	Human herpes virus 3 (varicella-zoster)
	Betaherpesvirinae	
	Cytomegalovirus	Human herpes virus 5 (CMV)
	Roseolovirus	Human herpes virus 6 and 7
	Gammaherpesvirinae	
	Lymphocryptovirus	Human herpes virus 4 (EBV)
	Rhadinovirus	Human herpes virus 8 (KSHV)
Polyomaviridae	*Polyomavirus*	JC, BK virus
Papillomaviridae	*Papillomavirus*	Human papillomavirus (HPV)
Ss DNA viruses	*Parvovirinae*	
Parvoviridae	*Erythrovirus*	B19

From: Gupta RK. In: *Pathology of opportunistic infections in tropics*. Jaypee; 2007

Herpetic Esophagitis in an Immunocompromised Patient

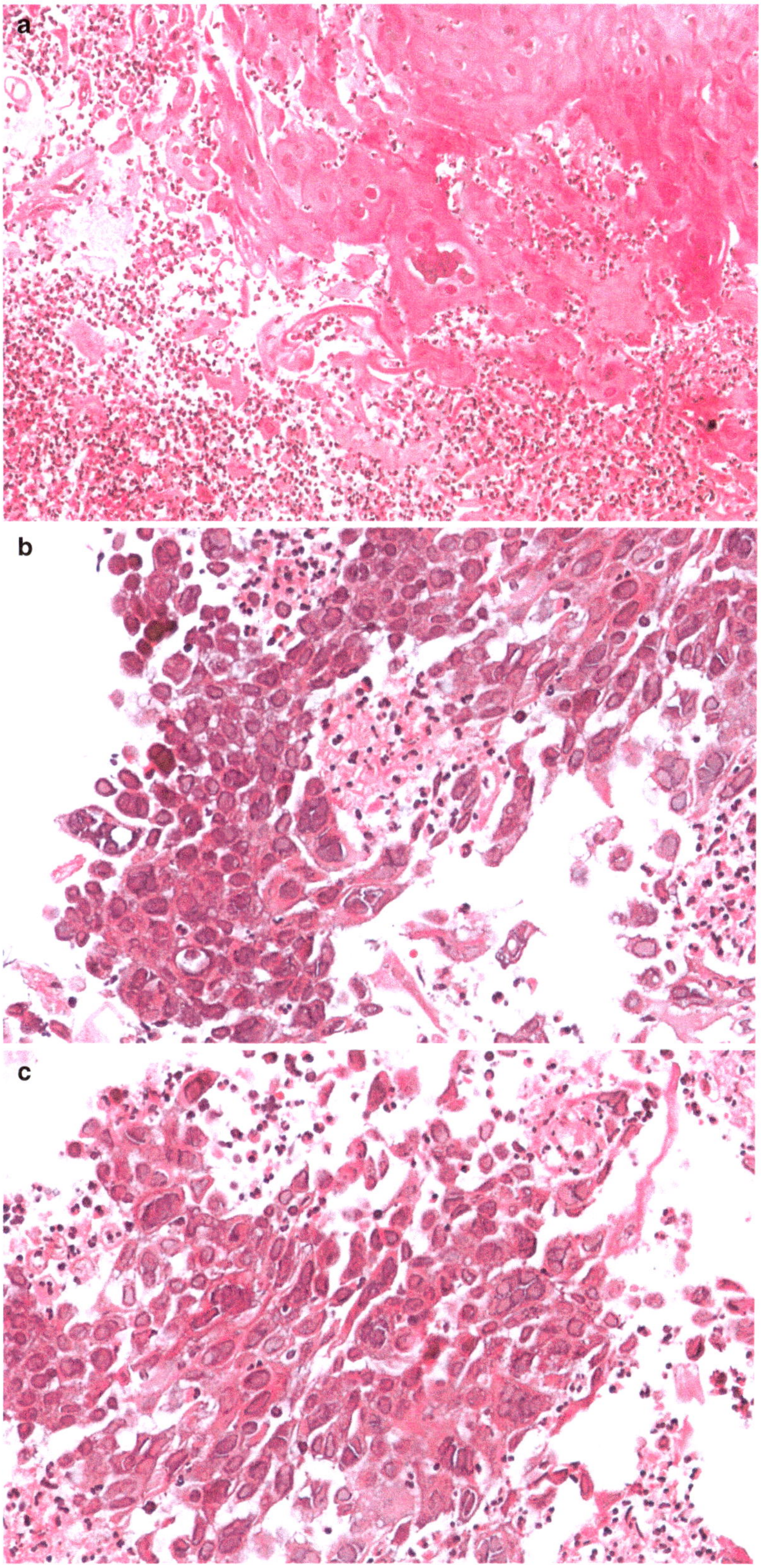

Fig. 3.1 (**a–c**) A 43-year-old female patient a known case of ulcerative colitis on long-term steroids, presented with dysphagia; there was no significant weight loss. Upper GI endoscopy showed multiple ulcers in lower esophagus. Laboratory workup revealed hemoglobin of 10.1 g/dl, TLC 9800/cu mm with neutrophils 61, lymphocytes 30, eosinophils 2, and monocytes 7 %, respectively. The platelet count was 233,000/cu mm. Histopathological examination of the endoscopic esophageal biopsy from ulcerated area revealed herpetic esophagitis (**a** HE ×200, **b**, **c** HE ×400)

Cytomegalovirus (CMV): CMV is an opportunistic pathogen and may produce persistent lifelong infection. It can be transmitted both vertically and horizontally through blood transfusion, sexual contact, and transplanted organs and from mother to the neonate by placenta, by cervicovaginal canal during child birth, or even through breast milk. Fetal transmission is seen in 20–30 % CMV-infected pregnant women.

In immunocompromised patients the severity of CMV disease correlates with the degree of immunosuppression. CMV-infected patients are known to develop superinfection with other pathogens like bacteria and fungi.

Tissue biopsy from the involved organ shows cytomegaly and nucleomegaly with the presence of characteristic intranuclear inclusions (Cowdry type A) in epithelial and/or endothelial cells. These inclusions are single, homogenous, and round to oval with smooth outline and appear amphophilic to basophilic in HE-stained sections. Intracytoplasmic inclusions may also be present. They are small, multiple, irregular, granular, and basophilic and are usually present in perinuclear zone; they are PAS and GSM positive. Immunohistochemistry performed on paraffin sections enhances the sensitivity of histological diagnosis.

Immunocompromised patients are unable to mount prompt immune response; hence, serodiagnosis may be inconclusive. PCR has replaced the cell culture as "gold standard" for CMV detection.

CMV Esophagitis in a Renal Allograft Recipient

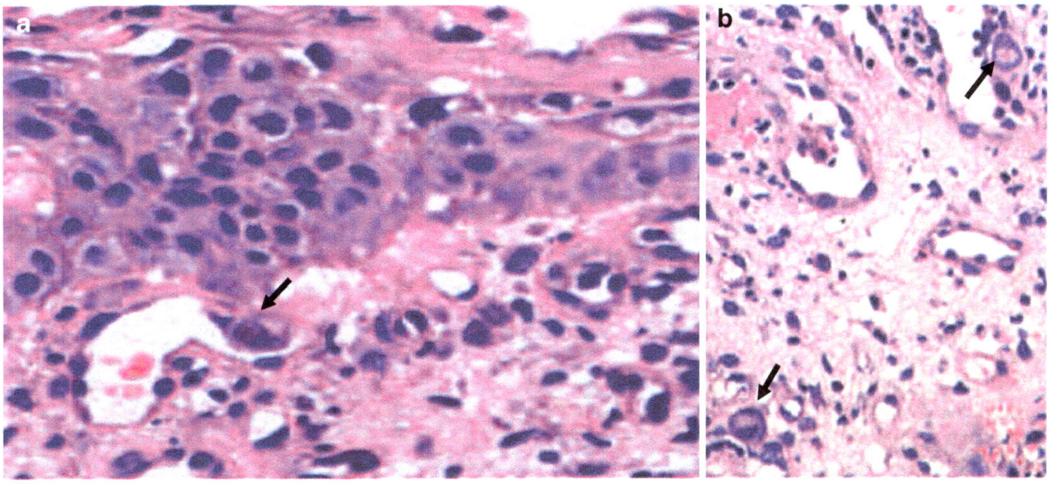

Fig. 3.2 (**a**, **b**) A-48-year-old male patient receiving live-related renal allograft presented 3 months posttransplant with complaints of epigastric discomfort. Upper GI endoscopy revealed mucosal hyperemia of the esophagus with the presence of edema and multiple linear ulcers. Biopsy from the ulcer showed inflammatory infiltrate; endothelial cells lining the capillaries showed marked cytomegaly and nucleomegaly and prominent eosinophilic intranuclear inclusions (*arrows*) suggestive of CMV esophagitis (**a** HE ×200, **b** HE ×400)

CMV Duodenitis in a Renal Allograft Recipient

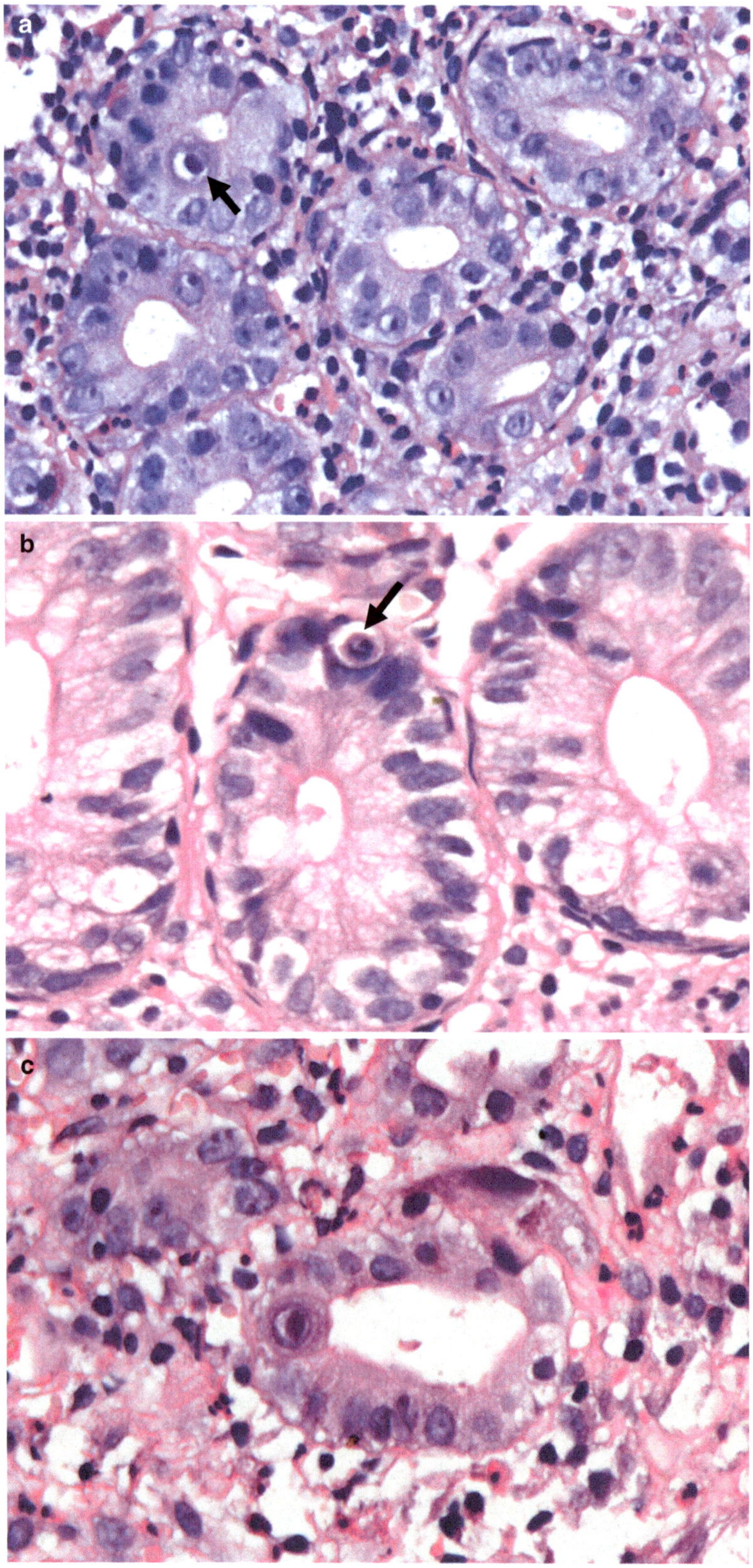

Fig. 3.3 (**a**–**d**) A-53-year-old male patient who received live-related renal allograft 10 years ago, presented with nausea and vomiting for 20 days. At admission to the hospital, his hemoglobin was 10.4 g/dl, and the serum creatinine was 3.31 mg/dl. TAC level was high; therefore, tacrolimus dose was reduced. Upper GI endoscopy revealed duodenal erosion. Duodenal biopsy showed that some of the glandular epithelial cells had nucleomegaly with intranuclear inclusions giving an owl eye appearance (*arrows*) suggestive of CMV duodenitis (**a**–**d** HE ×400)

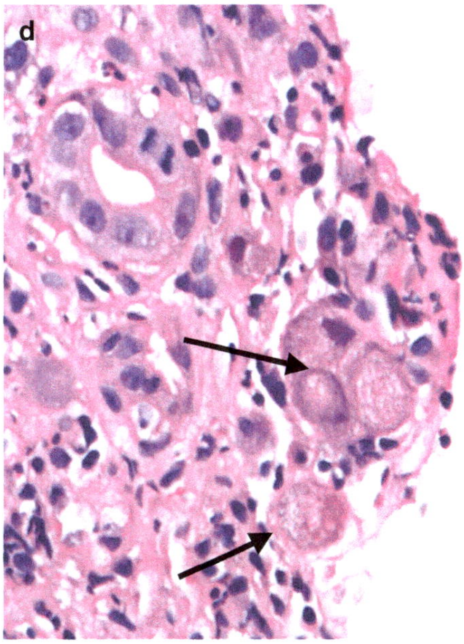

Fig. 3.3 (continued)

CMV Gastritis in a HIV-Positive Patient

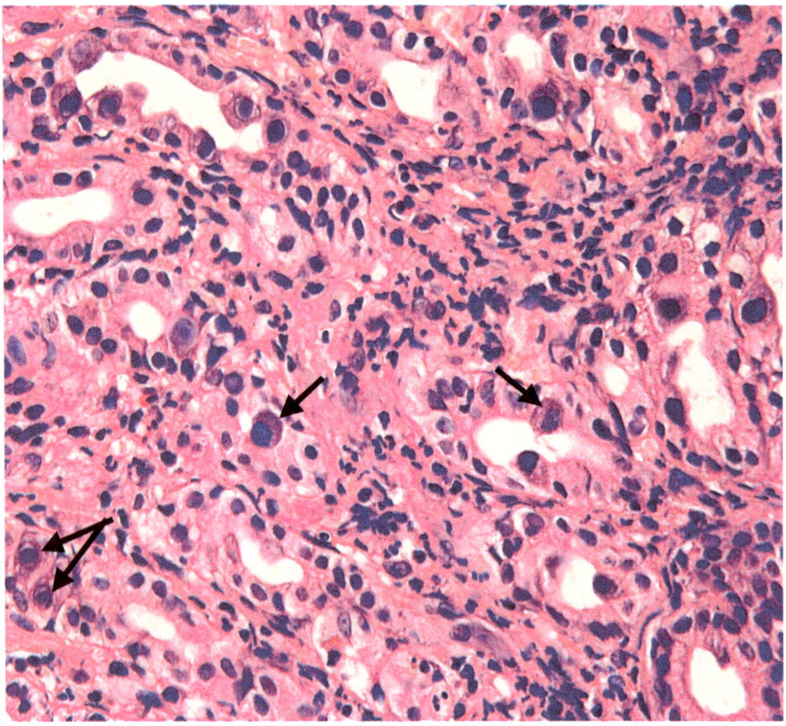

Fig. 3.4 A 56-year-old female patient with history of blood transfusion from a professional donor for ovarian surgery 8 years back presented with increased frequency of stools, large volume of watery diarrhea, occasional vomiting, loss of weight, and fever. Upper GI endoscopy revealed nodularity in the upper esophagus and stomach. Gastric biopsy showed mucosal ulceration along with cytomegaly and nucleomegaly with the presence of intranuclear "owl eye" inclusions in the glandular epithelial and endothelial cells (*arrows*), diagnostic of CMV gastritis (HE ×400). On subsequent investigations, the patient was found to be HIV positive with absolute CD4 count of 138/cu mm

CMV Colitis in Renal Allograft Recipient

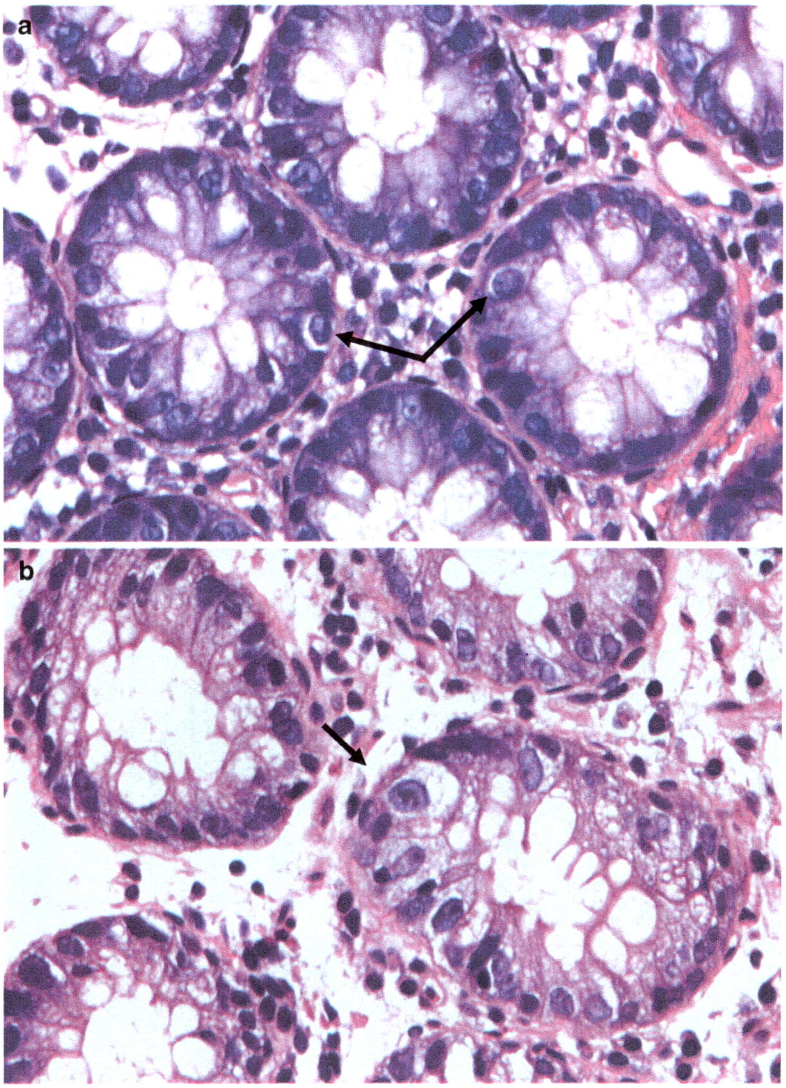

Fig. 3.5 (**a**, **b**) A 40-year-old male patient who received live renal allograft 7 years back and was maintained on triple drug immunosuppression, presented with persistent loose motions, weakness, and loss of weight for 3 months. His hemoglobin at admission was 9.1 g/dl; other lab parameters were within normal limits. Upper GI endoscopy did not reveal any abnormality; however, lower GI endoscopy showed multiple ulcers throughout the colon and sigmoid; multiple punch biopsies were obtained. The histological examination showed that some of the glandular epithelial cells had nucleomegaly with intranuclear inclusions giving an owl eye appearance (*arrows*) suggestive of invasive CMV colitis (**a**, **b** HE ×400). CMV PCR was positive

CMV Lung Disease in a HIV-Positive Patient

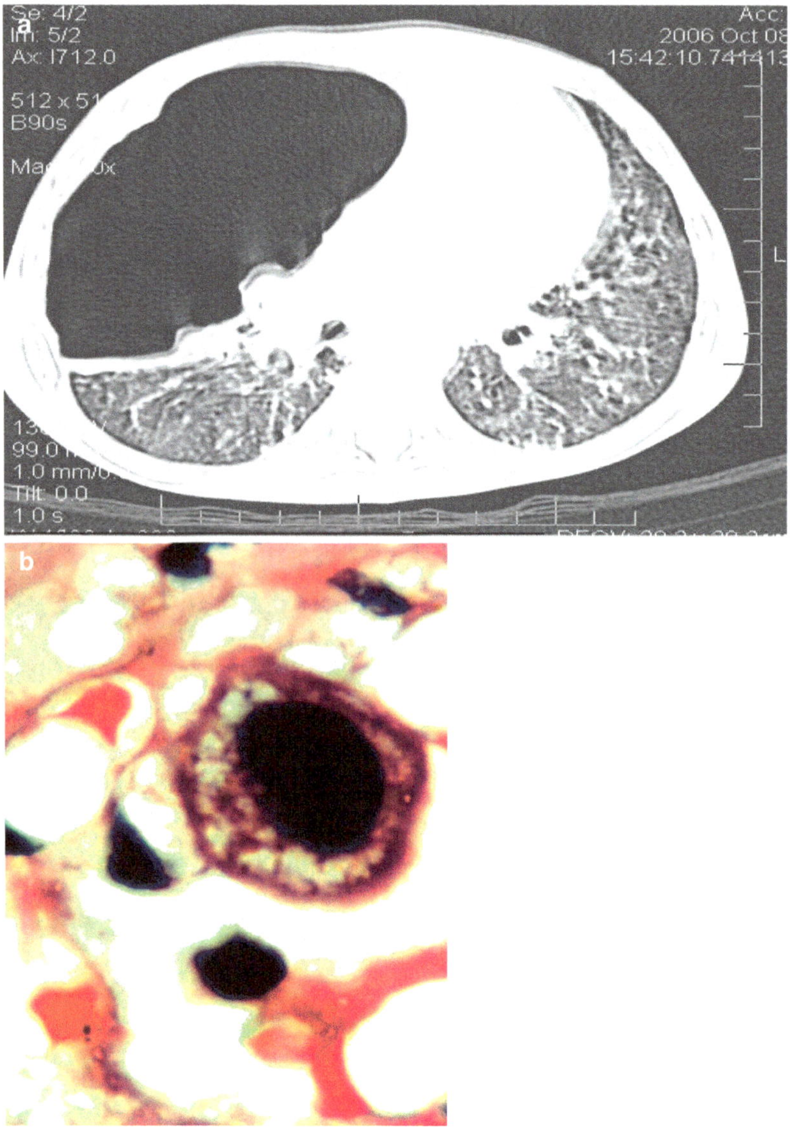

Fig. 3.6 (**a**, **b**) A 6-year-old male child presented with breathlessness for 4 months with fever and loss of weight for 1 month. The patient was HIV positive and was on retroviral therapy. Both parents were also HIV positive. CT chest revealed large cavity in the upper lobe of right lung with mass effect on the lower lobe with diffuse lung disease (**a**). Lobectomy of the upper lobe of right lung was performed. Histological examination of the resected lobe of the lung revealed that at places lining alveolar cells showed cytomegaly and nucleomegaly along with intranuclear owl eyelike inclusions suggestive of CMV lung disease (**b** HE ×1000) (Contributors – S. Radha and Tameem Afroz, Aware Global Hospital, Hyderabad, India)

CMV Skin Disease in a Renal Allograft Recipient

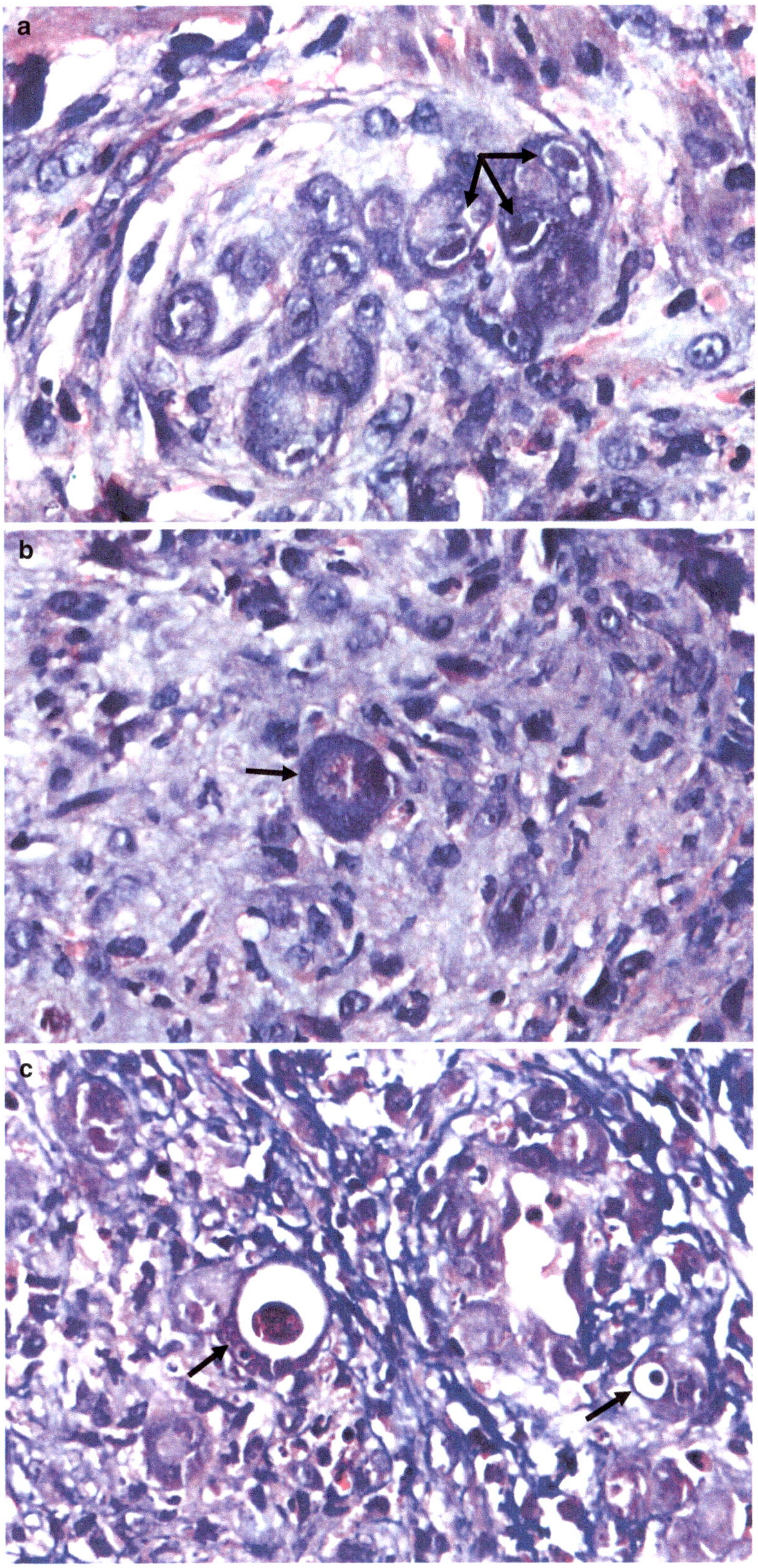

Fig. 3.7 (**a**–**c**) A 55-year-old male patient receiving spousal renal allograft was being maintained on triple drug immunosuppression. He developed posttransplant diabetes mellitus for which he received insulin. Three months later, he presented with multiple vesicular eruptions over the right axilla, scrotum, and penile skin for 6 weeks followed by fever for 2 weeks. His serum creatinine was 2.51 mg/dl, and he was anemic with a hemoglobin level of 5.6 g/dl. The patient had polymorphonuclear leukocytosis, total WBC count being 24,500/cu mm with 83 % neutrophils. Skin biopsy from the axillary ulcers revealed massive nucleomegaly with intranuclear owl eyelike inclusions (*arrows*) diagnostic of CMV disease in several vascular endothelial cells (**a**–**c** HE ×400)

CMV Disease in Fetus

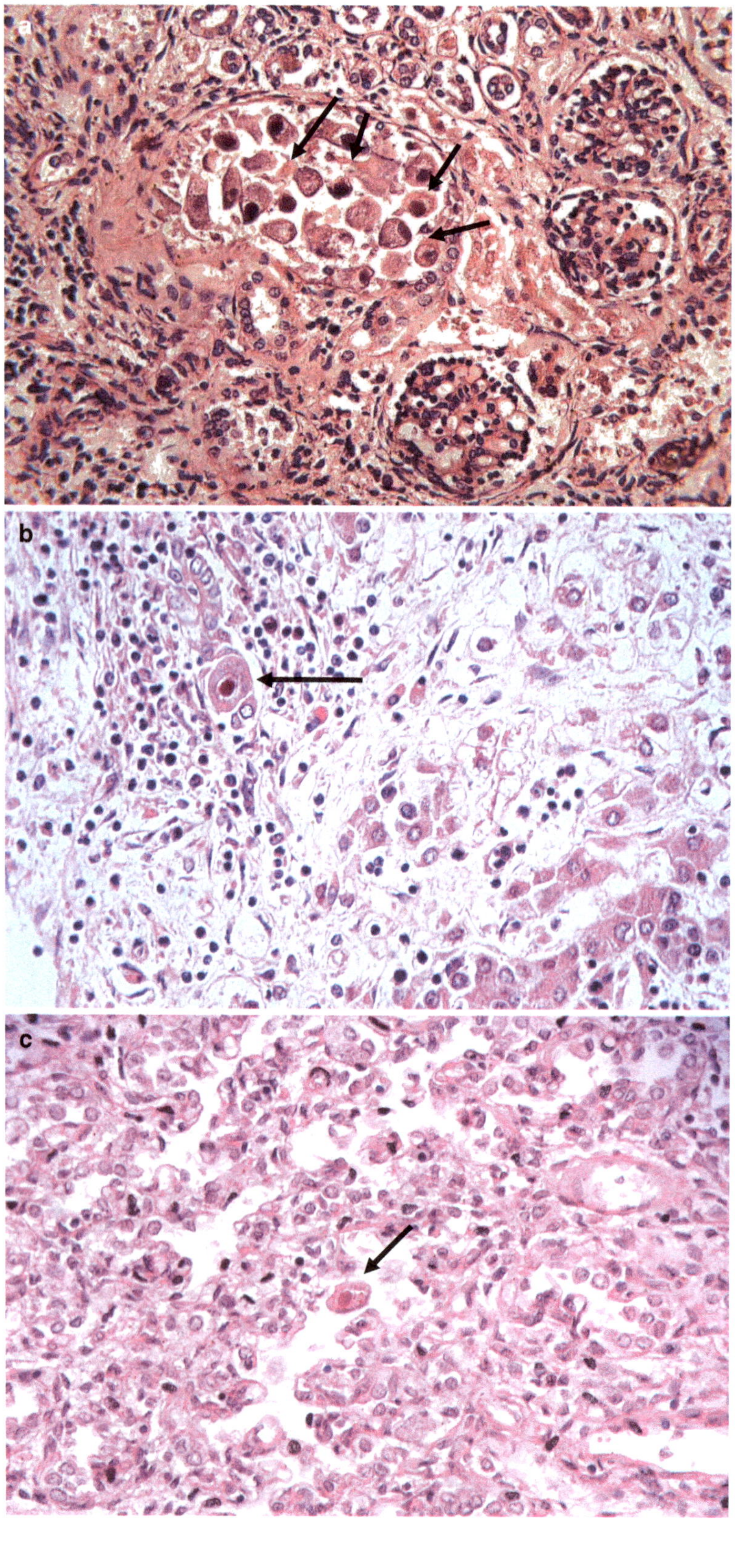

Fig. 3.8 (**a–c**) A 21-year-old primigravida delivered a stillborn fetus at 30 weeks of gestation. Fetal autopsy revealed massive hepatosplenomegaly with ascites. Provisional diagnosis of inborn errors of metabolism with hydrops fetalis was considered. Histopathological examination of both the kidneys showed fair number of tubular epithelial cells bearing intranuclear owl eyelike inclusions (**a** HE ×400). Immunohistochemistry with anti-CMV antibody showed positive staining in the cells showing nuclear inclusions. Sections from the liver and lungs also showed similar intranuclear inclusions in ductal and alveolar epithelial cells (**b**, **c** HE ×400). HIV status of fetus or parents was not known (Contributor – Prof. Vinita Agrawal, Department of Pathology, Sanjay Gandhi Postgraduate Institute of Medical Sciences, Lucknow, India)

Polyomavirus: JC and BK viruses are the important members of this group. They share 75% homology at the nucleotide sequence level. They are opportunistic pathogens causing disease in immunocompromised conditions including AIDS, renal transplant and bone marrow transplant, immunosuppressive drug therapy, granulomatous diseases, and autoimmune states such as rheumatoid arthritis and SLE.

BK virus may cause nephropathy in renal transplant recipients; these patients show interstitial nephritis mimicking organ rejection. Viral inclusions may be seen in tubular epithelial cells. IHC is useful in demonstration of viral antigen on paraffin sections.

BKV Nephropathy in a Renal Allograft Recipient

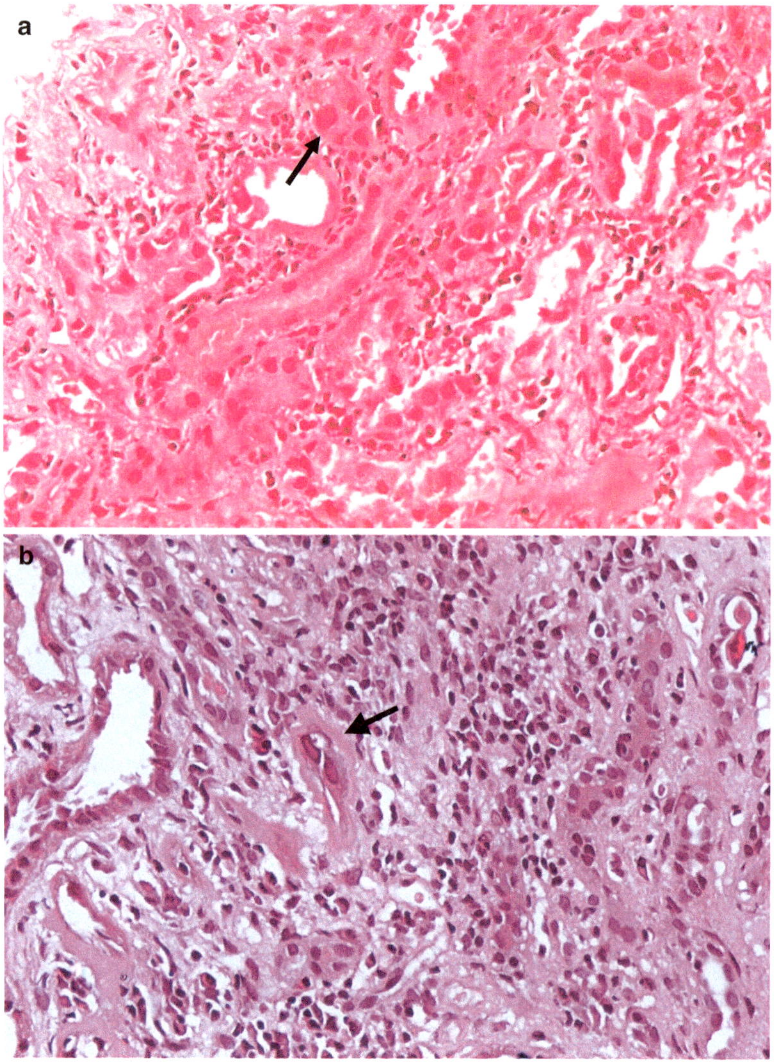

Fig. 3.9 (**a**–**c**) A 55-year-old male patient receiving spousal renal allograft was being maintained on triple drug immunosuppression consisting of prednisolone, tacrolimus, and MMF. He developed new-onset diabetes after transplantation (NODAT). After 5 months of transplantation, he presented with acute graft dysfunction; serum creatinine was 1.6 mg/dl against baseline of 1.1 mg/dl; serum tacrolimus C2 level was 5 ng/ml. Doppler ultrasound of the graft kidney was found to be within normal limits. Serology for CMV, HSV1, and HSV2 was negative. Renal allograft biopsy showed tubulointerstitial nephritis with presence of mild tubulitis. Some of the endothelial and tubular epithelial cells showed markedly enlarged nuclei with intranuclear inclusions (*arrow*). Immunohistochemistry for SV 40 antigen was positive suggesting BK virus nephropathy (**a** HE ×400, **b** PAS ×400 and **c** IHC ×400)

Fig. 3.9 (continued)

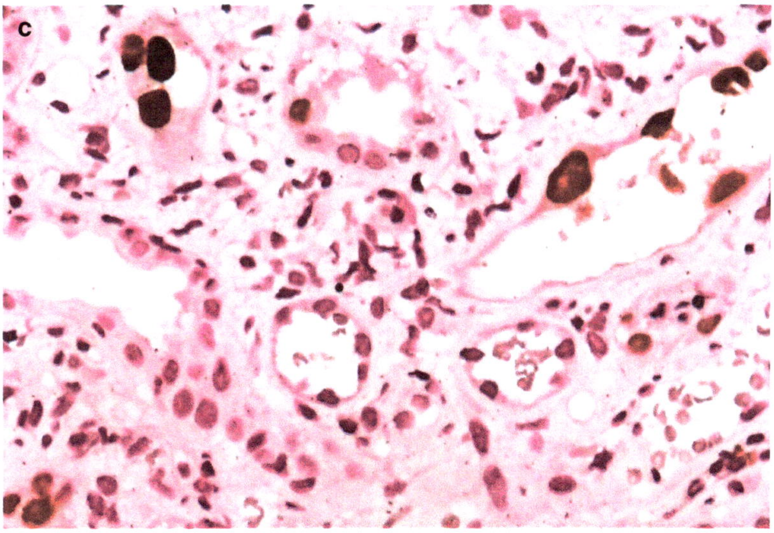

Molluscum Contagiosum in an Immunocompromised Patient

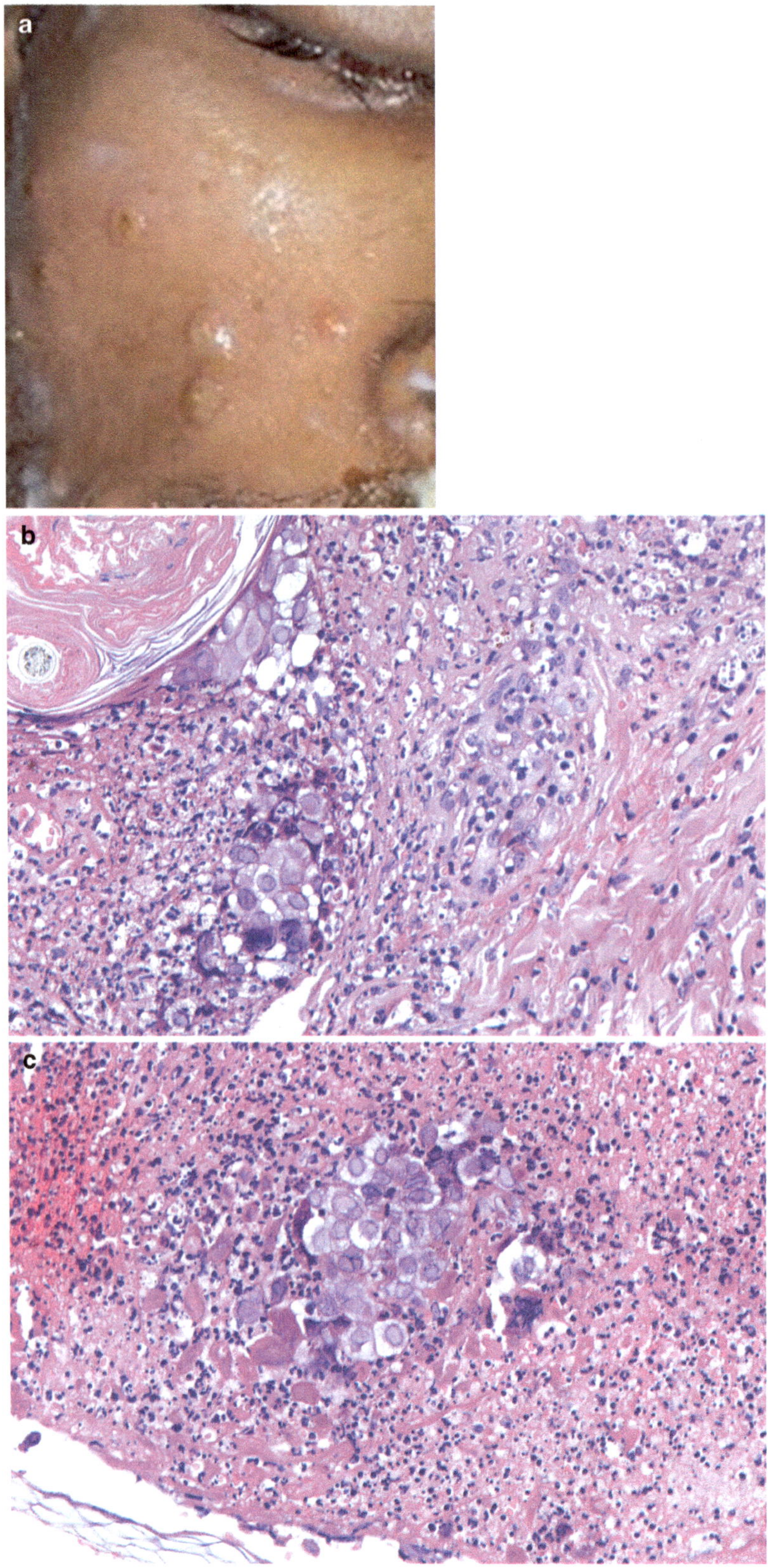

Fig. 3.10 (**a–d**) A 22-year-old male patient presented with high fever for 4 days. There was no organomegaly; however, he was hypotensive. Laboratory workup revealed a total WBC count of 33,400/cu mm with 95 % neutrophils and shift to left. The total serum proteins were 4.47 g/dl with albumin of 2.72 g/dl, serum creatinine was 5.5 mg/dl, and serum urea was 145 mg/dl. SGOT was 104 IU/L and SGPT was 289 IU/L. Serum calcium was 6.07 mg/dl with ionized calcium of 0.76 mg/dl. Serum procalcitonin was >200 ng/ml and PTH was 403.10 pg/ml; serum amylase was also high (463.9 U/L). *Acinetobacter* was grown on blood culture. Eleven days after hospitalization, he developed umbilicated lesions on his face (**a**). Serology for HIV was negative. Skin biopsy from the lesion showed epidermal cells containing large intracytoplasmic inclusions called "molluscum bodies"; the nucleus of the cell was pushed to the periphery. Tissue necrosis with acute inflammatory response was evident around ruptured molluscum bodies (**b**, **c** HE ×200, **d** PAS ×200)

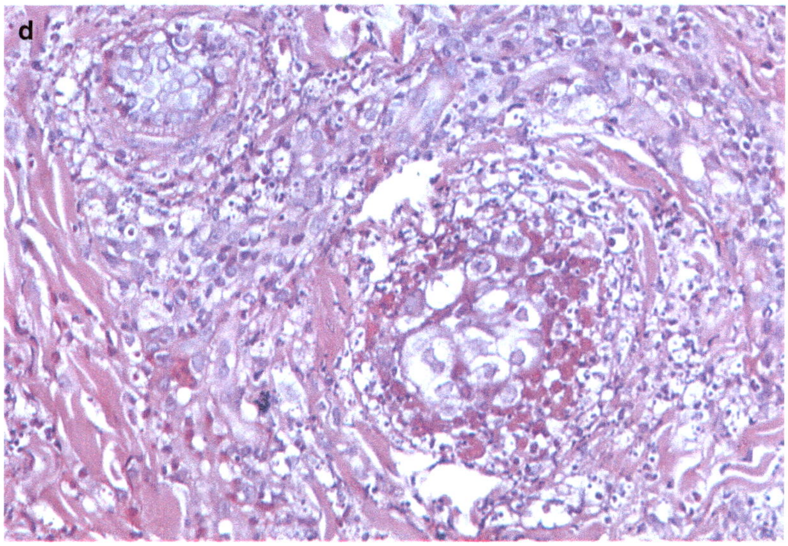

Fig. 3.10 (continued)

Papillomavirus: Human papillomavirus (HPV) infects stratified squamous epithelium of man and is associated with various benign lesions such as warts, cervical intraepithelial neoplasia, and squamous cell carcinoma of cervix. Patients with immunocompromised states such as lymphoma and HIV infection and organ transplant recipients are at increased risk of developing cutaneous warts. The risk of developing anogenital warts increases 10–100-folds in renal allograft recipients and fourfold in HIV-infected patients. The risk increases with increasing number of sexual partners. Cervical and oral cancers associated with HPV have also been found in patients on immunosuppressive therapy including allograft recipients. Viral antigen can be demonstrated on paraffin sections by IHC.

Condyloma Acuminatum in a Renal Allograft Recipient

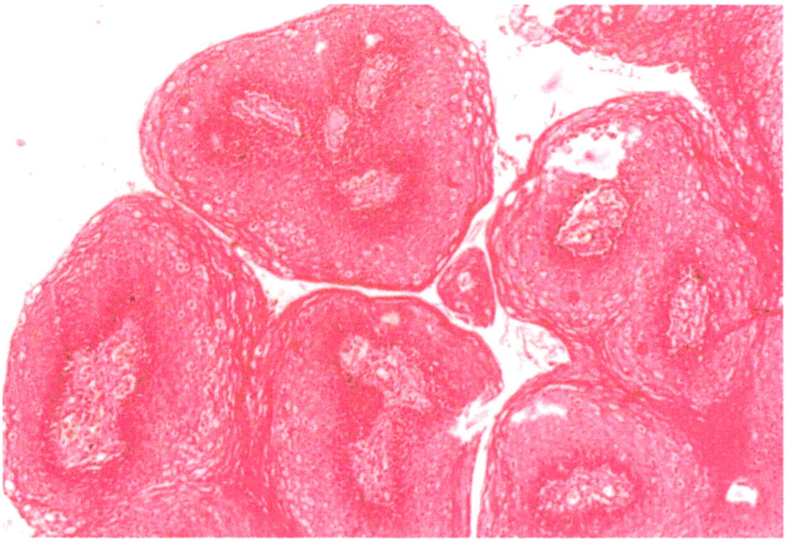

Fig. 3.11 A 40-year-old male patient who received live-related renal allograft presented 6 years posttransplant with a cauliflower-like growth on the glans penis. Histopathological examination revealed condyloma acuminatum. Thereafter, he presented with multiple recurrences of similar lesions on the scrotum and penis (HE ×100) (From: *Pathology of Opportunistic Infections in Tropics*, Jaypee; 2007)

Epstein-Barr Virus (EBV): EBV is widespread with a seroprevalence of 80–90 %. Unregulated EBV proliferation in patients with impaired cell-mediated immunity such as AIDS and allograft recipients on immunosuppressive therapy commonly leads to EBV-associated lymphoproliferative neoplasms.

PTLD of the Kidney in a Renal Allograft Recipient

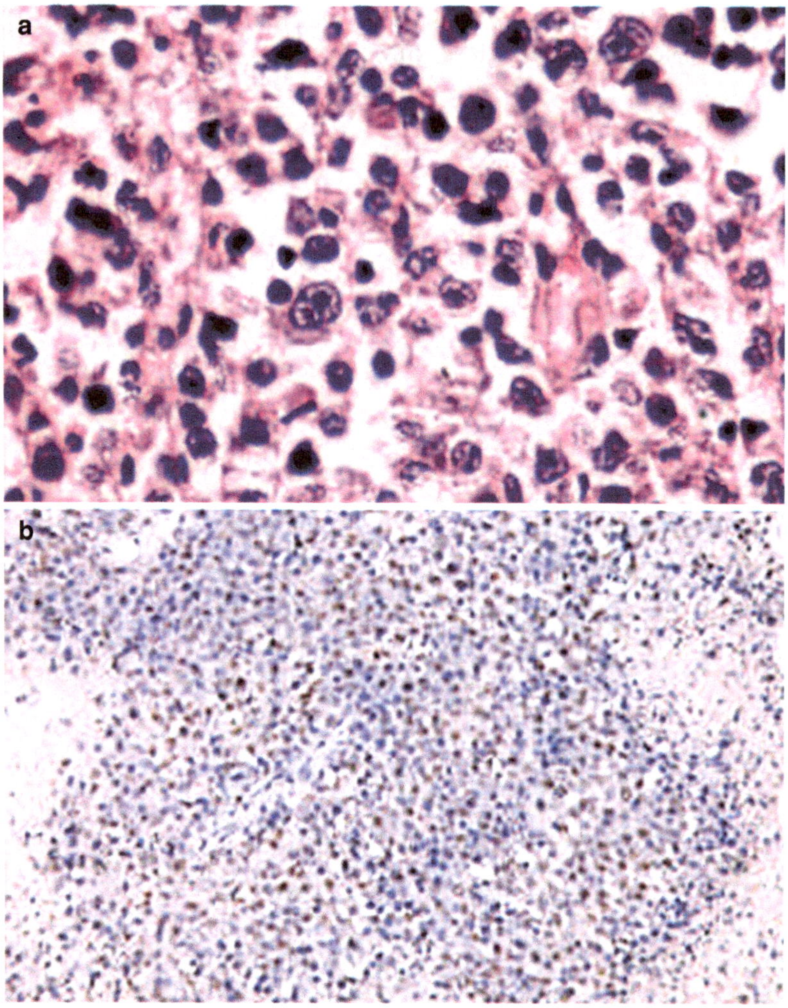

Fig. 3.12 (**a–d**) A 30-year-old male patient who received live-related renal allograft; 3 years posttransplant presented with high-grade fever with loss of weight and appetite. CT abdomen revealed a lobulated mass at hilum of transplanted kidney with heterogeneous density and areas of cystic change. Graft nephrectomy was performed. Histological evaluation of the hilar mass and graft nephrectomy specimen revealed that the hilar mass consisted of large atypical lymphoid cells diffusely infiltrating and replacing renal parenchyma (**a** HE ×400). Immunohistochemistry for EBV Zebra antigen and lambda and kappa light chains was suggestive of EBV-associated monoclonal high-grade B-cell posttransplant lymphoproliferative disorder (PTLD) (**b** IHC for Zebra, **c** lamda, and **d** kappa antigens ×200) (Contributor – Prof. Kusum Joshi, Department of Histopathology, Postgraduate Institute of Medical Education and Research, Chandigarh, India) (From: Gupta RK. In: *Pathology of Opportunistic Infections in Tropics*, Jaypee; 2007)

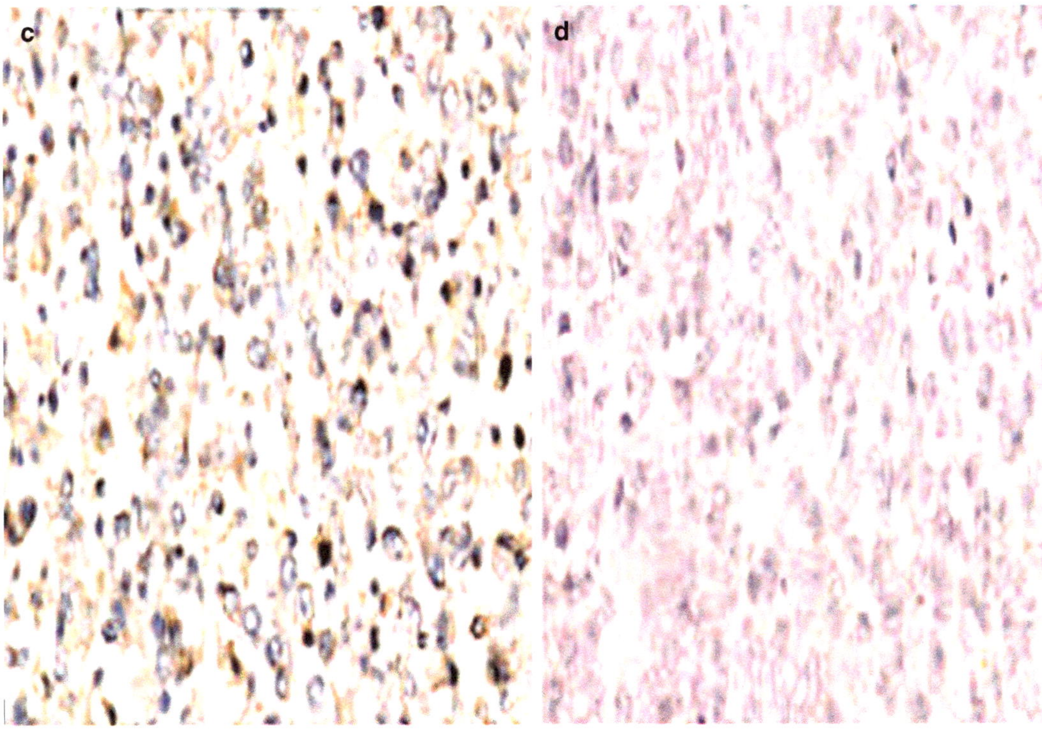

Fig. 3.12 (continued)

Hodgkin-Like PTLD in an Allograft Kidney

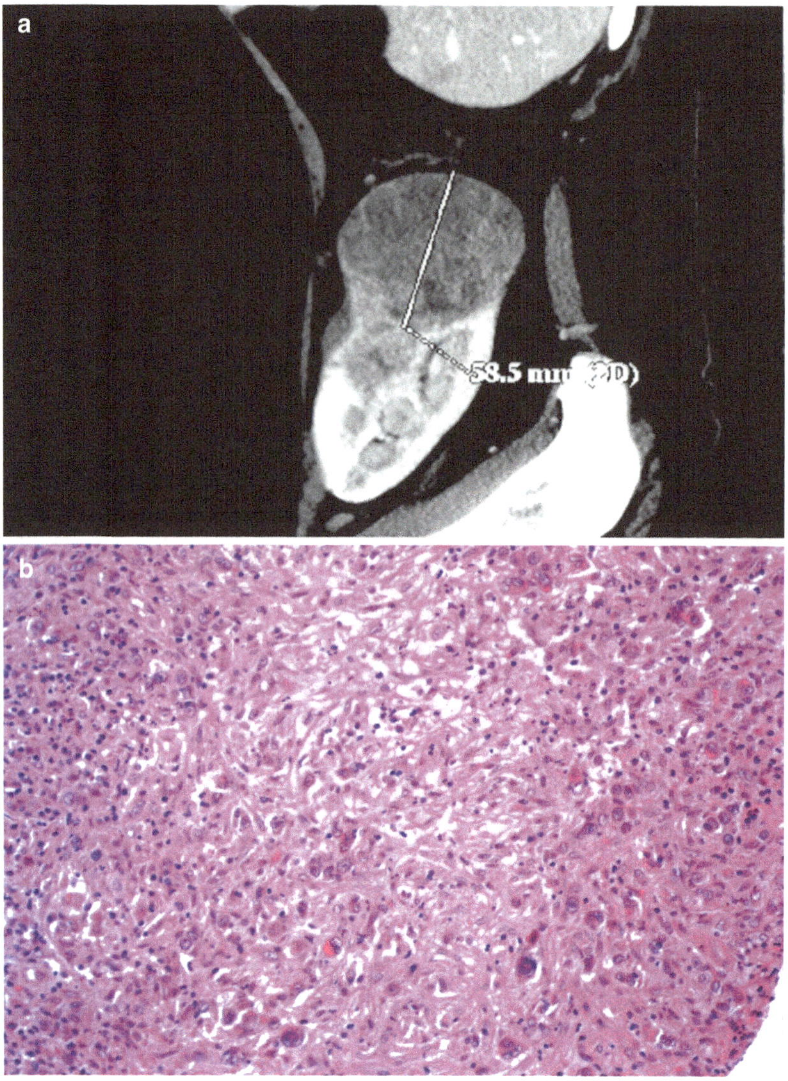

Fig. 3.13 (**a**–**h**) A 25-year-old female patient receiving live-related renal allograft (donor mother) 10 years posttransplant presented with loss of weight and appetite for 3 months. CT lower abdomen showed a SOL in the upper pole of the allograft kidney (**a**). Needle core biopsy of the mass showed a polymorphic infiltrate with many Hodgkin cells and few multinucleate forms suggestive of Hodgkin-like PTLD (**b** HE ×200, **c**–**h** IHC showing the large cells strongly positive for CD30, CD15, focal positivity for CD20, and dim nuclear positivity with PAX5) (Contributor – Swarnalata Gowrishankar, Senior Consultant Pathologist, Apollo Hospitals, Jubilee Hills, Hyderabad, India)

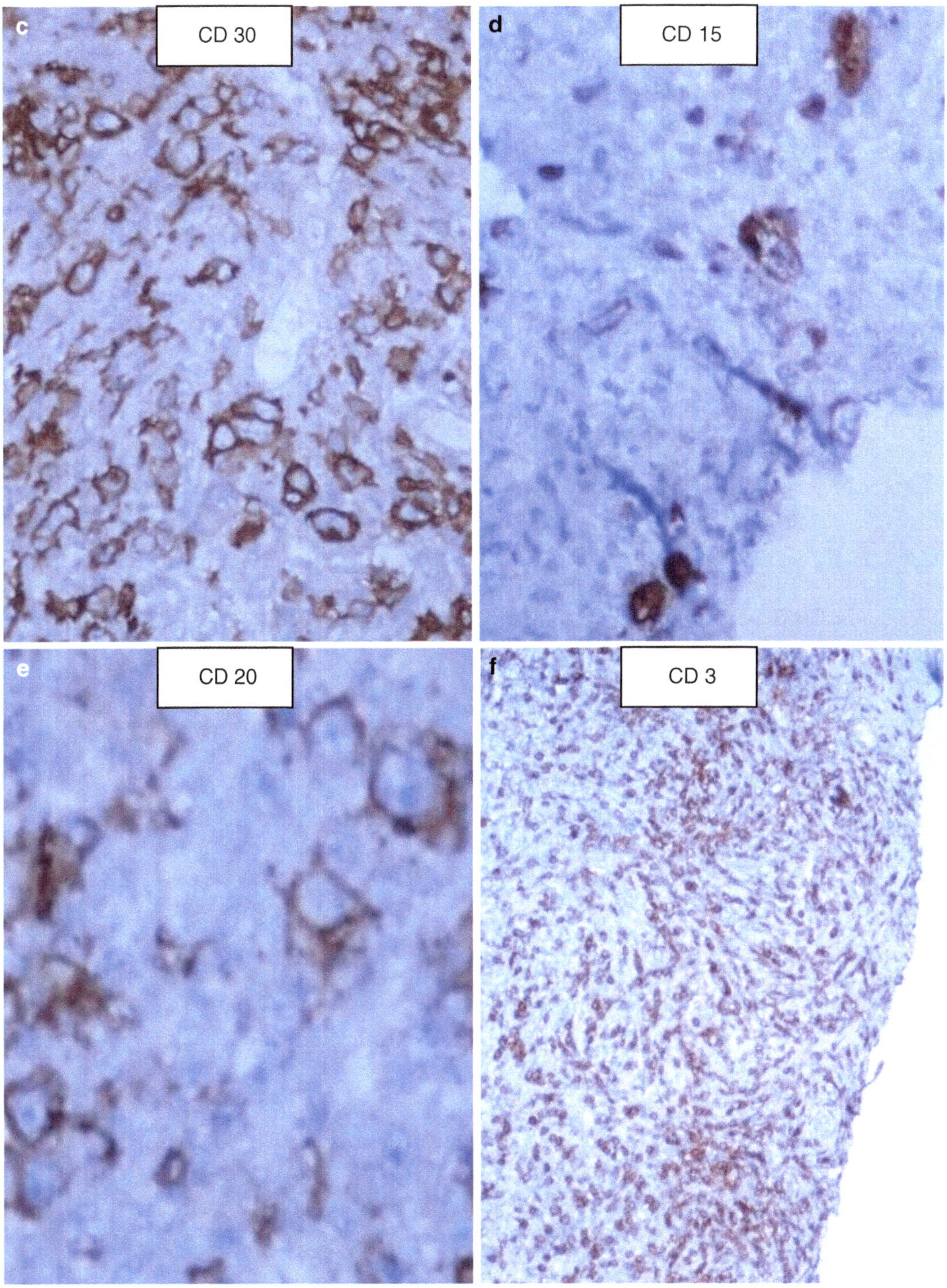

Fig. 3.13 (continued)

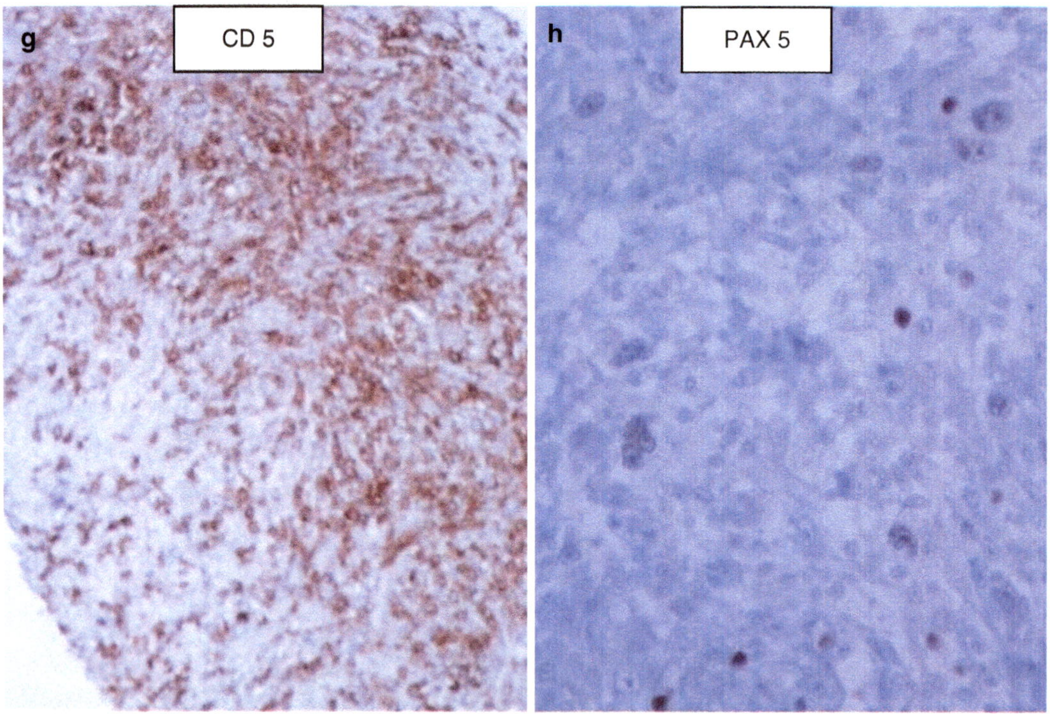

Fig. 3.13 (continued)

PTLD of the Testis with Skin Involvement in a Renal Allograft Recipient

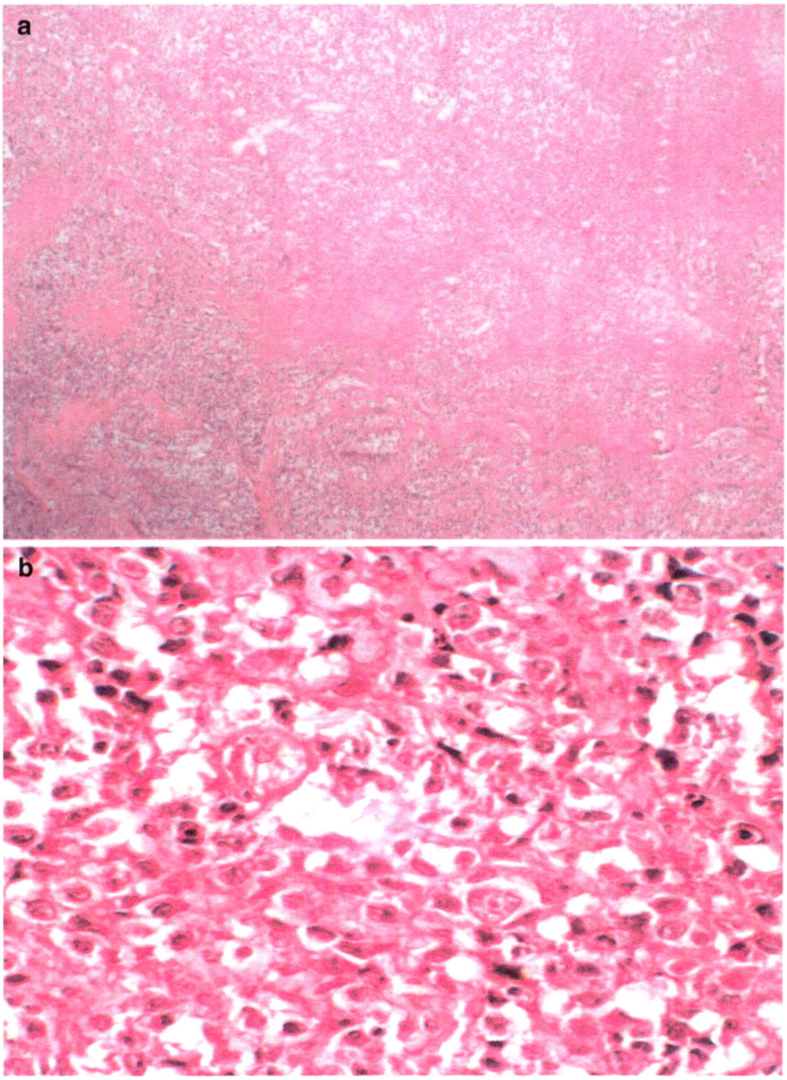

Fig. 3.14 (**a**–**e**) A 31-year-old male patient received live-related renal allograft in 1993, and he was maintained on triple drug immunosuppression. Posttranplant period was uneventful. Seven years later, he presented with fever and pain in left inguinoscrotal region. Clinical examination revealed that the left testis was swollen and tender; subsequently he developed scrotal ulceration. Left orchidectomy with debridement of scrotal skin was performed. Histological examination of testis and cutaneous lesion revealed monomorphic diffuse large B- cell lymphoma (PTLD) (**a** HE ×100, **b** HE ×400; **c** HE ×200, **d**–**f** IHC ×400) (Contributor – Prof. Manoj Jain, Department of Pathology, Sanjay Gandhi Postgraduate Institute of Medical Sciences, Lucknow, India)

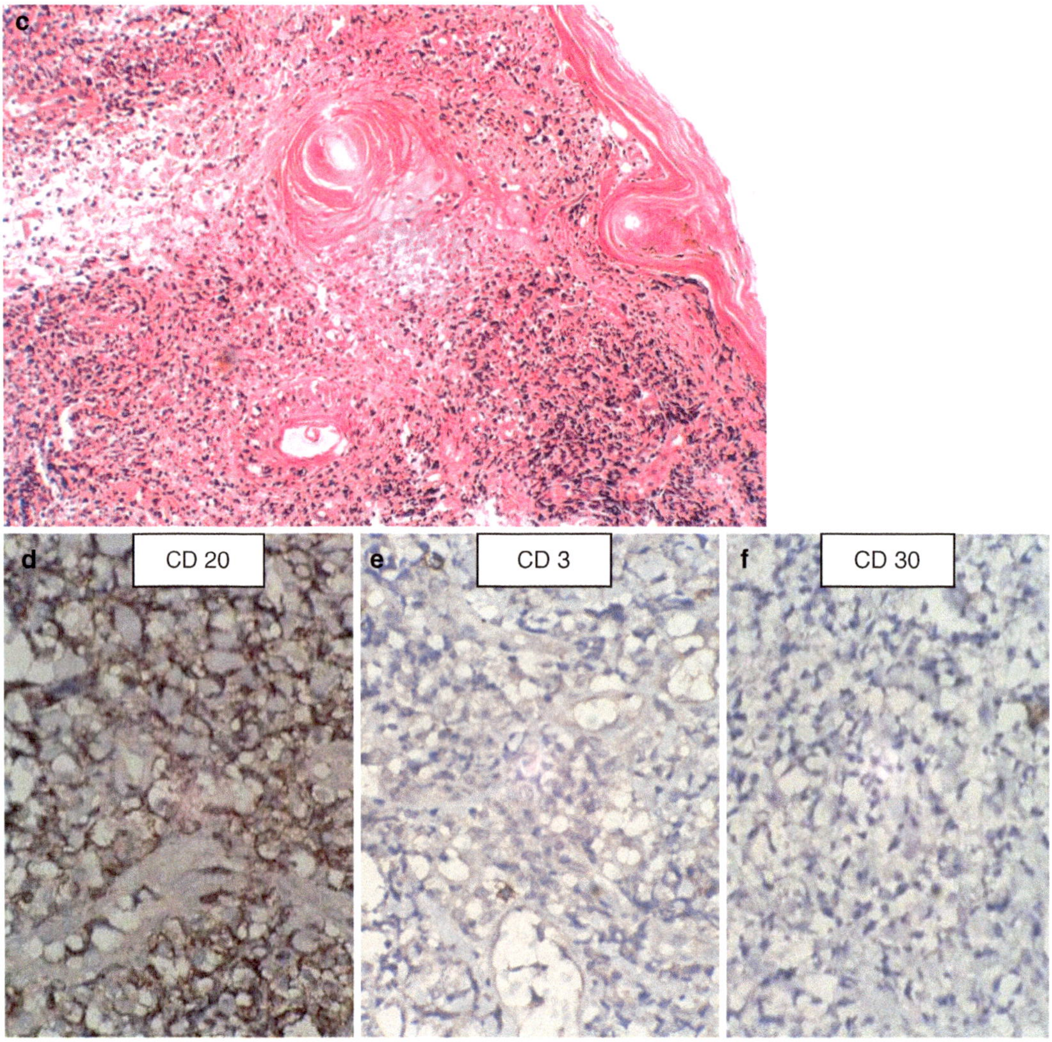

Fig. 3.14 (continued)

PTLD of the DJ Junction in a Renal Allograft Recipient

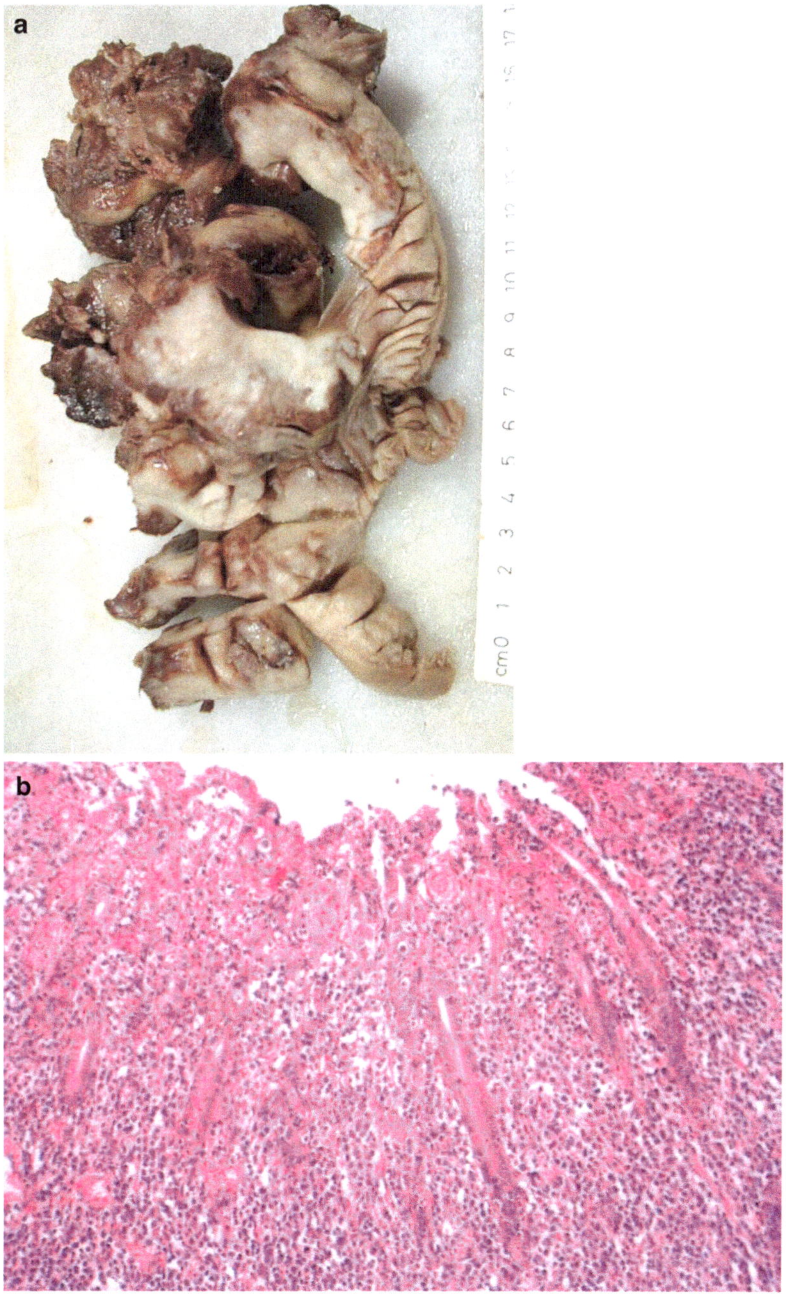

Fig. 3.15 (**a**–**e**) A 31-year-old male patient received live-related renal allograft in 1993, and he was maintained on triple drug immunosuppression. Posttranplant period was uneventful. Eight years later, he presented with gastric outlet obstruction. Upper GI endoscopy revealed narrowing of DJ junction. CT revealed mass in D3, D4, and jejunum. EBV serology was negative. Bone marrow examination did not show any lymphomatous infiltration. Surgical resection of a loop of DJ region with mass was performed. Histological examination revealed monomorphic diffuse large B-cell lymphoma (PTLD) (**a** gross specimen, **b** HE ×200, **c** HE ×400, **d**, **e** IHC ×400) (Contributor – Prof. Manoj Jain, Department of Pathology, Sanjay Gandhi Postgraduate Institute of Medical Sciences, Lucknow, India)

Fig. 3.15 (continued)

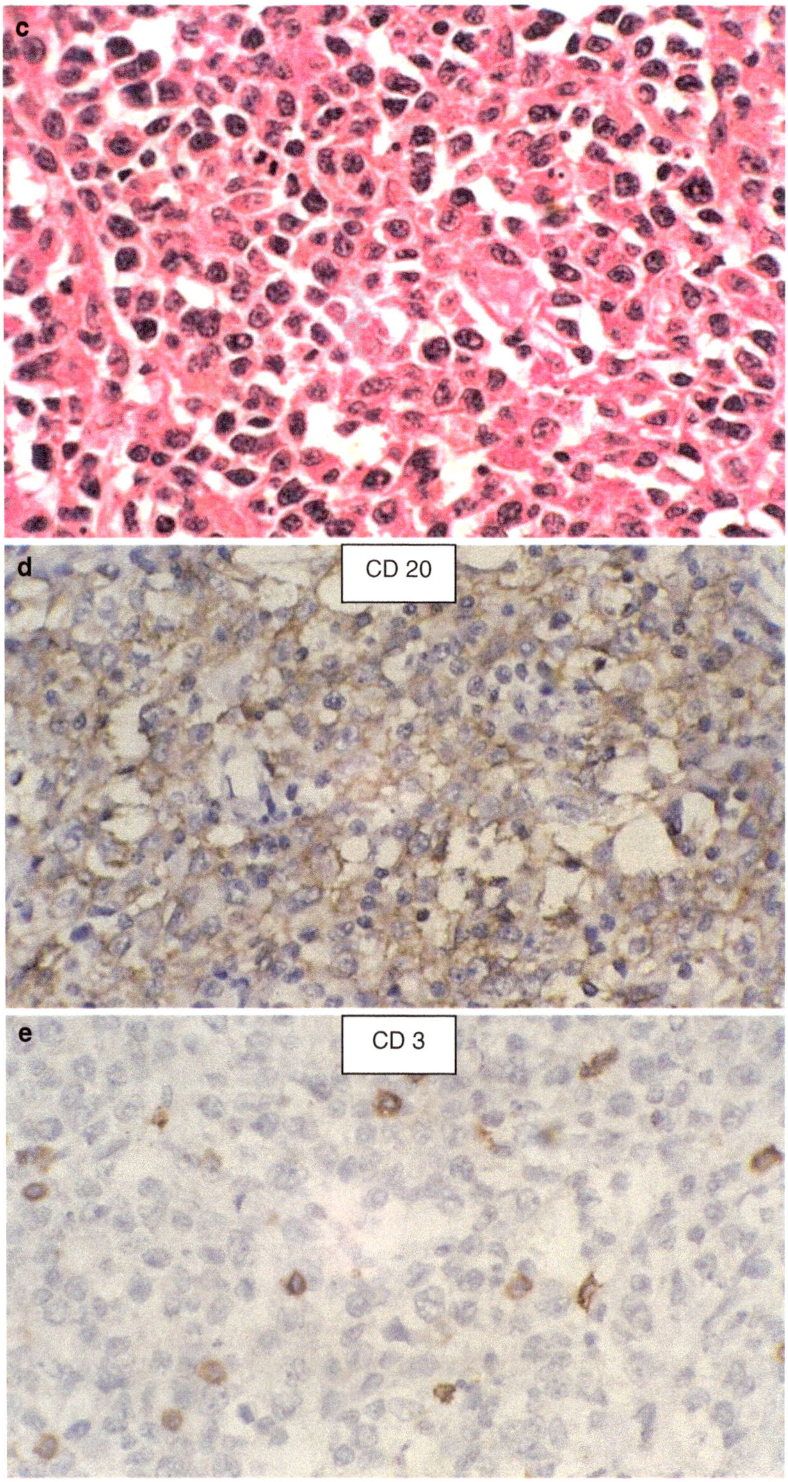

PTLD of the Jejunum in a Renal Allograft Recipient

Fig. 3.16 (**a**–**i**) A 28-year-old male patient received live-related renal allograft in October 1998. He was maintained on triple drug immunosuppression. Posttransplant period was uneventful. Five years later, he presented with anemia and hematochezia for 15 days followed by abdominal pain and vomiting for 1 day. Clinical examination revealed a soft lump in the lower abdomen. Exploratory laparotomy showed a large growth in the jejunum. Histological examination revealed monomorphic diffuse large B-cell lymphoma (PTLD) (**a**, **b** gross specimen, **c** HE ×100, **d** HE ×200, **e**, **f** HE ×400, **g**–**i** IHC ×200) (Contributor – Prof. Manoj Jain, Department of Pathology, Sanjay Gandhi Postgraduate Institute of Medical Sciences, Lucknow, India)

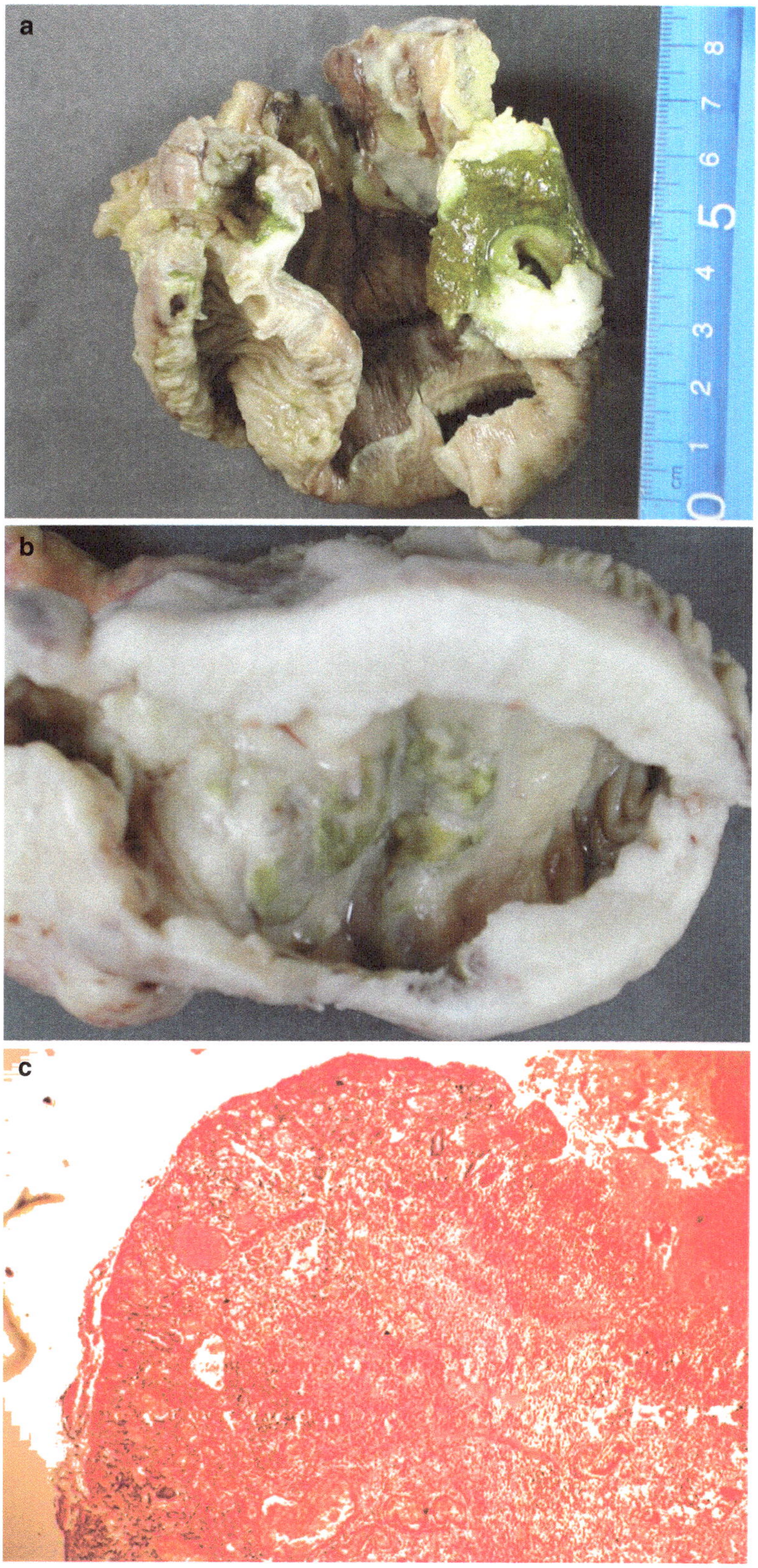

Fig. 3.16 (continued)

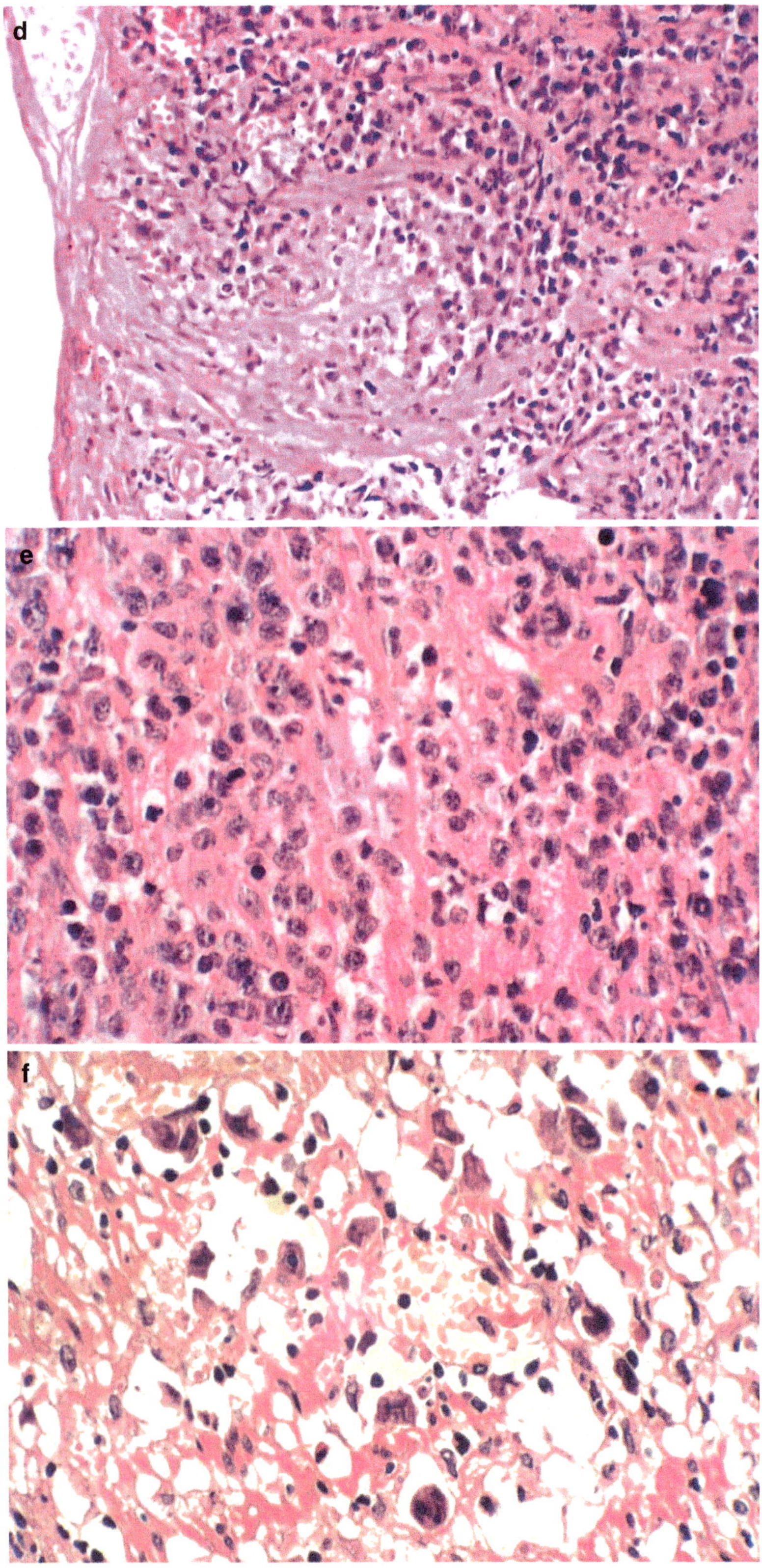

Fig. 3.16 (continued)

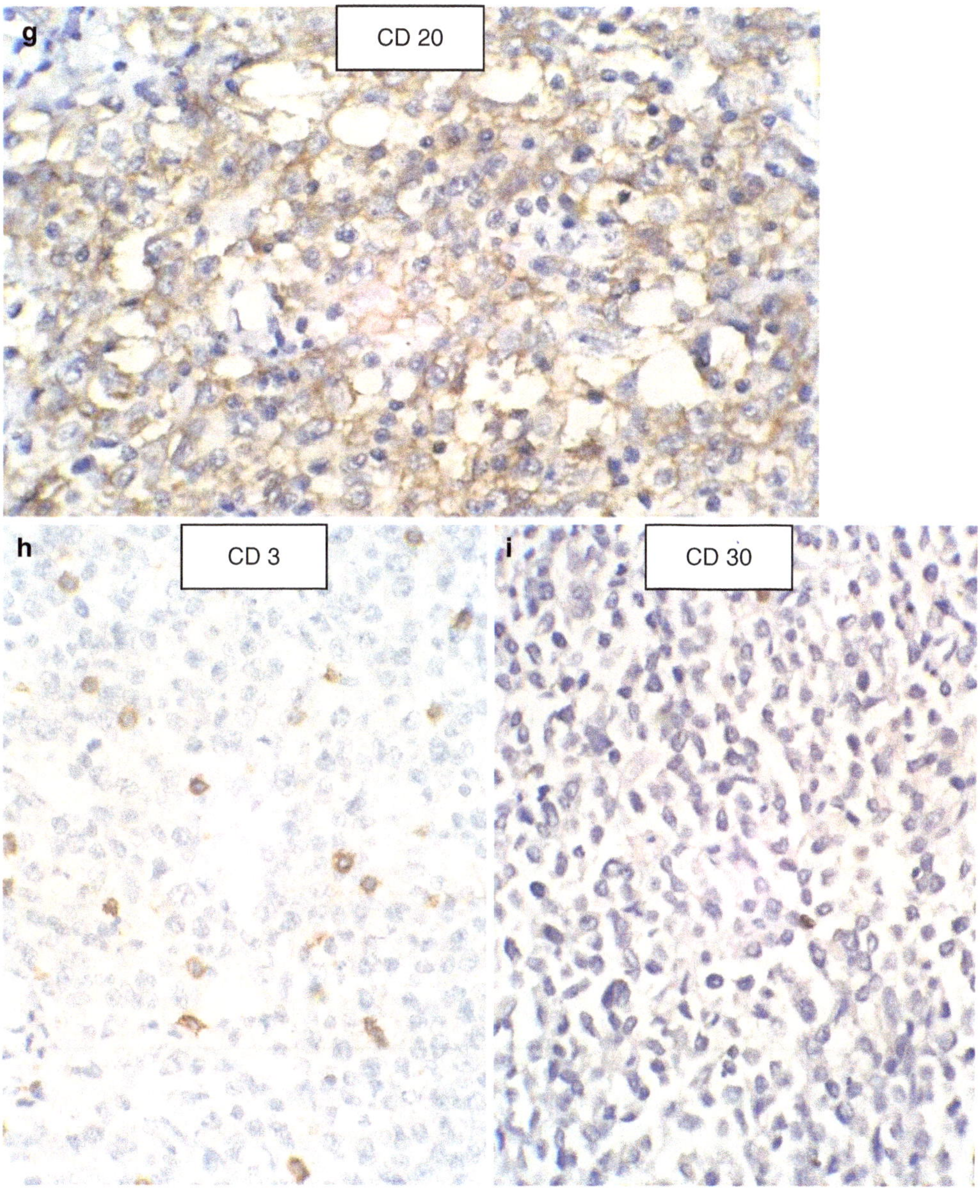

PTLD of the Lymph Node and Liver in a Renal Allograft Recipient

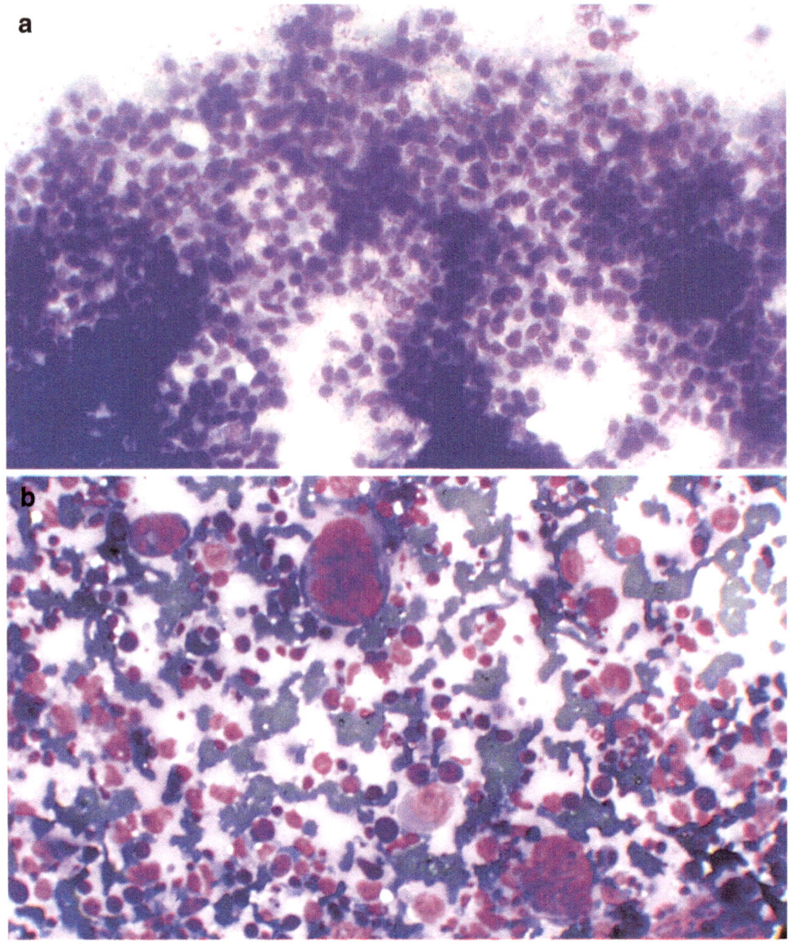

Fig. 3.17 (**a**, **b**) A 36-year-old male patient received live-related renal allograft in March 1994 and was maintained on triple drug immunosuppression. Ten years posttransplant, he presented with low-grade pyrexia, anorexia, abdominal pain, epigastric burning, altered bowel habits, and vomiting for 1 month. USG abdomen showed lymphadenopathy. USG-guided FNA revealed high-grade NHL (**a** MGG ×200). Three months later, he developed a nodule in the liver; USG-guided FNA from liver SOL also showed similar morphology (**b** MGG ×200). The patient received chemotherapy and died 4 months later (Contributor – Prof. Manoj Jain, Department of Pathology, Sanjay Gandhi Postgraduate Institute of Medical Sciences, Lucknow, India)

Fig. 3.18 (**a**–**c**) A 10-month-old male infant (full-term low birth weight, normal vaginal delivery) presented with high-grade fever for 10 days followed by 3 episodes of generalized tonic-clonic seizures. Subsequently the patient developed bilateral cervical lymphadenopathy, generalized maculopapular rash, hematemesis, and melena. His weight was 7.5 kg, height 71 cm, and the head circumference 41 cm. He had mild pallor and healed mucosal ulcers in the oral cavity. Liver span was 4.5 cm below the right costal margin in midclavicular line with rounded borders and coarse echotexture on USG. Spleen was enlarged 4.0 cm below the left subcostal margin. Upper GI endoscopy did not reveal any abnormality. The laboratory workup revealed hemoglobin content of 9.7 g/dl, total leukocyte count of 37,000/cu mm with 71 % lymphocytes, and presence of activated lymphoid cells in the peripheral blood smear. Plasma fibrinogen was low (122 mg/dl) and serum ferritin was high (822 μg/L). Liver function tests revealed that the serum bilirubin was 1.2 mg/dl (conjugated 0.7 mg/dl), total serum proteins were 6.4 g/dl with serum albumin of 2.4 g/dl. Hepatic enzymes were raised (SGOT 131 U/L, SGPT 105 U/L, GGT 802 U/L, and LDH 695 U/L). EBV, HAV, HBV, HCV, and HIV serology were negative. PCR showed amplification for parvovirus genomic sequences. Bone marrow aspiration and bone marrow biopsy showed giant proerythroblasts (**a** Leishman stain ×400); some of these cells contained intranuclear eosinophilic inclusions with peripheral chromatin condensation (*arrows*) (**b** Leishman stain ×400) along with giant proerythroblast with prominent nucleoli and cytoplasmic blebs (*dog ears cytoplasm*) considered diagnostic of parvovirus infection (**c** Leishman stain ×1000). Liver biopsy showed mild nonspecific steatohepatitis

Parvovirus Infection (Fifth Disease) in an Infant

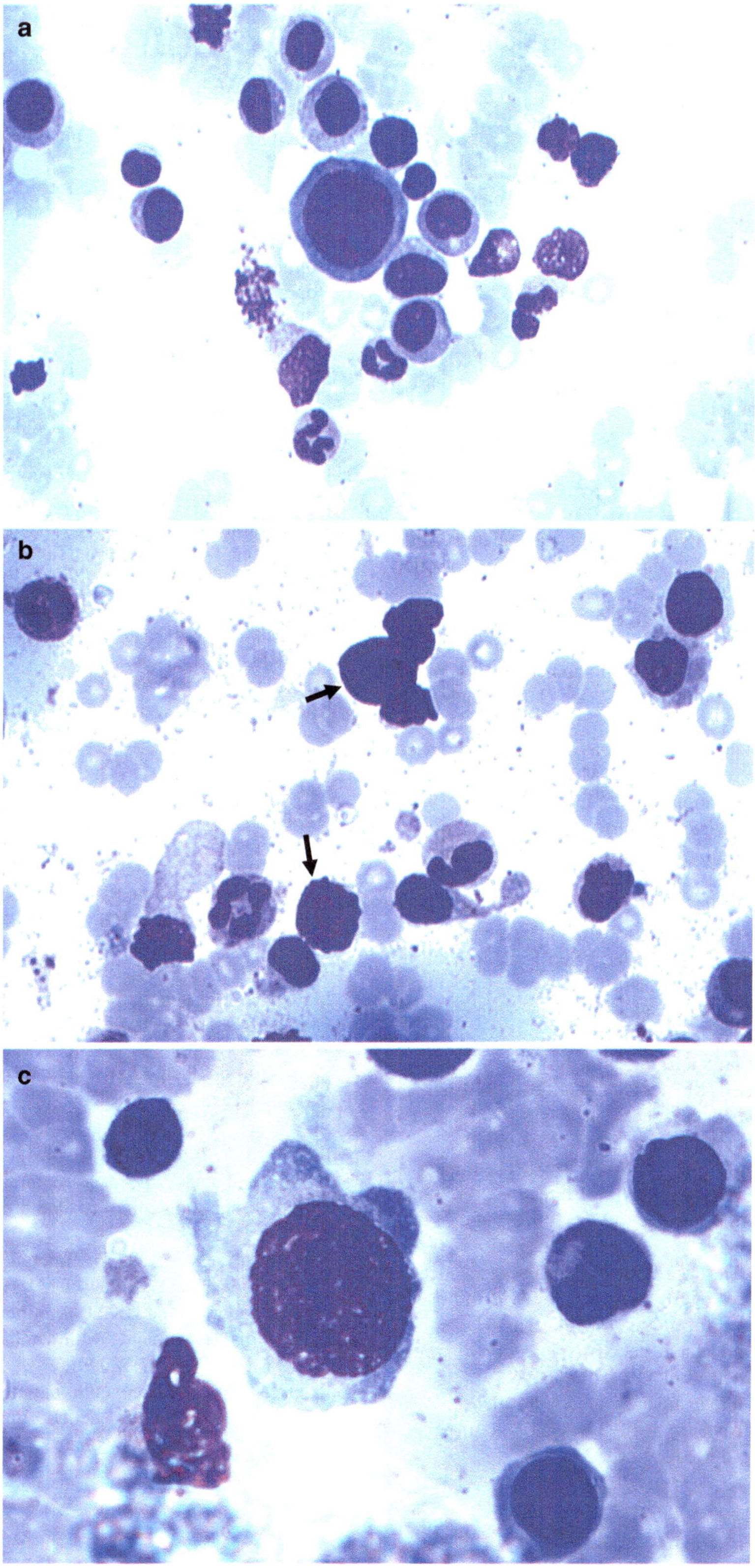

Further Reading

1. Agrawal V, Gupta RK, Jain M, Prasad N, Sharma RK. Polyomavirus nephropathy and Cytomegalovirus nephritis in renal allograft recipients. Indian J Path Microbiol. 2010;53:672–5.
2. Alford C. Breast milk transmission of cytomegalovirus (CMV) infection. Adv Exp Med Biol. 1991;310:293–7.
3. Anagnostopoulos I, Hummel M, Finn T. Heterogenous E-B virus infection patterns in peripheral T-cell lymphoma of angioimmunoblastic lymphadenopathy type. Blood. 1992;80:1804–12.
4. Andres D, Hassan AF, Walker P, Sweny GPD, Emery VC. Prospective study of human beta herpes viruses after renal transplantation: association of hhv-7 and CMV coinfection with CMV disease and increased rejection. Transplantation. 2000;69:2400–4.
5. Balfeur HH. Varicella zoster virus infection in 1C hosts. A review of the natural history and management. Am J Med. 1988;85:68–73.
6. Berger T, Sawchuk WS, Leonardi C, et al. Epidermodysplasia verruciformis – associated papillomavirus infection complicating human immunodeficiency virus. Br J Dermatol. 1991;124:79–83.
7. Berneman ZN, Ablashi DV, Li G et al. Human herepes virus 7 is a T lymphotropic virus and is related to, but significantly different from human herpes virus 6 and human cytomegalovirus. Proc Nalt Acad Sci. 1992;89:10552–6.
8. Bosch FX, Manos MM, Munoz N, Shernan M, Jansen AM, Peto J, Schiffman MH, Moseno V, Kurman R, Shah KV. International biological study on cervical cancer (IBSCC) study group: prevalence of human papillomavirus in cervical cancer: a worldwide perspective. J Natl Cancer Inst. 1995;87:796–802.
9. Boshoff C, Schultz TF, Kennedy MM, et al. Kaposi's sarcoma association – herpes virus infects endothelial and spindle cells. Nature Med. 1995;1:1274–8.
10. William B. BK polyomavirus: a newly recognized threat to transplanted kidneys. Clev Clin J Med. 2003;70:1056–68.
11. Chang Y, Cesarman E, Persun MS, Lee F, Culpepper J, Knowles DM, Moore PS. Identification of herpes virus like DNA sequences in AIDS – associated Kaposi's sarcoma. Science. 1994;265:1865–9.
12. Chen JH, Mao YY, He Q, Wu JY, Lv R. The impact of pretransplant cytomegalovirus infection on acute renal allograft rejection. Transplant Proc. 2005;37:4203–7.
13. Chesters PM, Heritage J, Mc Cance DJ. Persistence of DNA sequences of BK virus and JC virus in normal human tissues. J Infect Dis. 1983;47:676–84.
14. Enders G. Varicella-zoster virus infection in pregnancy. Prog Med Virol. 1984;29:166–96.
15. Evan AS, Subrahmanya L, et al. Prevalence, incidence and persistence of EB virus antibody in young adults. N Engl J Med. 1970;282:361–5.
16. Griffiths PD, Emery VC. Clinical and laboratory evaluation of CMV induced mononucleosis in previously healthy individuals: report of 82 cases. Medicine. 1986;65:124–34.
17. Gupta RK. Opportunistic infections in renal allograft recipients. Transplant Proc. 2007;39:731–3.
18. Gupta RK. Opportunistic viral infections. In: Pathology of opportunistic infections in tropics. New Delhi: Jaypee; 2007. p. 15.
19. Gutierrez J, Vergara MJ, Guerrero M, et al. Multiple sclerosis and human herpes virus 6. Infection. 2000;30:145–9.
20. Holman RC, Janssen RS, Buehler JW, Zelashy MT, Hooper WC. Epidemiology of PML in the United States: analysis of national mortality and AIDS surveillance data. Neurology. 1991;41:1733–6.
21. Hoshino K, Nishi T, Adachi H, et al. Human herpes virus 6 infection in renal allografts: retrospective immunohistochemical study in Japanese recipients. Transplant Int. 1995;8:169–73.
22. International Committee on Taxonomy of viruses. In: Regenmortel MHVran, Fauquet CM, Bishop DHL, et al, editors. Virus taxonomy. Seventh report of the International Committee on Taxonomy of viruses. San Diego: Academic Press, Inc.; 2000.
23. Jain M, Badwal S, Pandey R, Srivastava A, Sharma RK, Gupta RK. Post-transplant lymphoproliferative disorders in live donor renal transplantation. Clin Transplant. 2005;19:669–73.
24. Kunn L, Sun XW, Wright Jr TC. Human immunodeficiency virus infection and female lower genital tract malignancy. Cur Opin Obstet Gynecol. 1999;11:35–9.
25. Leigh IM, Buchanan JA, Harwood CA, Cerio R, Storey A. Role of human papilloma-viruses in cutaneous and oral manifestations of immunosuppression. J Acquir Immune Defic Syndr. 1999;21:549–57.
26. Lopez C, Honess RW. HHV-6. In: Fields BN, Knipe DM, editors. Virology. 2nd ed. New York: Raven; 1990. p. 2055–62.
27. Mattes M, McLaughtien JE, Emery VC, Clarck DA, Griffiths PD. Histopathological detection of owl's eye inclusions is still specific for CMV in the era of human herpes virus 6 & 7. J Clin Pathol. 2000;53:612–4.
28. Morey AL, Ferguson DJP, Lesle KO, Taatjes DJ, Fleming KA. Intracellular localization of parvovirus B19 nucleic acid at the ultrastructural level by in situ hybrid with digoxigenin – labeled probes. Histochem J. 1993;25:421–9.
29. Nickeleit V, Klimkait T, Buiet IF, Dahlquer P, Delzenero V, Thiel G, Mihatsch MJ, Hirsch H. Testing for polymavirus type BK DNA in plasma to identify renal allograft recipients with viral nephropathy. N Engl J Med. 2000;342:1309–15.
30. Palefxky JM. Human papillomavirus infection and anogenital neoplasia in human immunodeficiency virus-positive men and women. J Natl Cancer Inst. 1998;23:15–20.

31. Richman DD, Whitley RJ, Hayden FG. Virus in: clinical virology. Washington, DC: ASM Press; 2002. p. 447.
32. Richtsmeier WJ, Wittels EG, Mazur EM. Epstein–Barr virus-associated malignancies. Crit Rev Clin Lab Sci. 1987;25:105–36.
33. Rubin RH. Importance of the CMV in the transplant population. Transpl Infect Dis. 1999;1:3–7.
34. Salahuddin SZ, Ablashi DV, Markhan PD, Josephs SF, Sturzenegger S, Kaplan M, Halligan G, Biberfetd P, Wong Staal F, Kramarsk B. Isolation of a new virus, HBLV in patients with lymphoproliferative disorders. Science. 1986;234596–601.
35. Shibata D, Weiss L, Hernandez A, Nath WB, Bernstein L, Levine A. Epstein-Barr virus associated lymphoma in patients infected with the human immunodeficiency virus. Blood. 1993;81:2102–9.
36. Sillman FH, Sentovich S, Shaffer D. Anogenital neoplasia in renal transplant patients. Ann Transplant. 1997;2:59–66.
37. Stagno D, Pass RF, Cloud G, et al. Primary cytomegalovirus infection in pregnancy: incidence, transmission to fetus and clinical outcome. JAMA. 1986;256:1904–8.
38. Suga S, Yoshikawa T, Nagai T, Asano Y. Clinical features and virological findings in children with primary human herpes virus 7 infection. Pediatrics. 1997;99:e4.
39. Takanashi M, Ito M, Sakamoto F, Shimizu FT, Takahashi M, Matsunaga Y. Parvovirus B19 infection: immunohistochemical and electron microscopic studies of skin lesions. J Cutan Pathol. 1998;22:168–72.
40. Tieben LM, Berkhout RJ, Smits HL, et al. Detection of epidermodysplasia verruciformis like human papillomavirus types in malignant and premalignant skin lesions of renal transplant recipients. Br J Dermatol. 1994;131:226–30.

4 Opportunistic Fungal Infections

Opportunistic fungal infections cause considerable morbidity and mortality in immunocompromised individuals including organ transplant recipients, patients with HIV/AIDS, and those receiving radiochemotherapy for various malignant lesions. Abrasions in cell-mediated immunity lead to deep mycoses in most of the cases; neutropenic patients may also develop invasive aspergillosis or deep candidiasis. Defects in humoral immunity do not predispose to fungal infections.

These infections are often rapidly progressive. Therefore, strong clinical suspicion and rapid, accurate, and prompt diagnosis of fungal infection are crucial for the initiation of prompt and appropriate antifungal therapy. Commonly encountered fungal infections in immunocompromised patients are listed in Table 4.1.

Candida Species (Causative Agent of Candidiasis): *Candida* species are ubiquitous yeasts and form normal flora of the skin and mucosa of alimentary, respiratory, and genitourinary tract. In immunocompromised patients, abrasions in host defense mechanisms result in tissue invasion of the fungus and causation of infection. The clinical manifestations could predominantly be cutaneous, mucocutaneous, or disseminated candidiasis with deep organ involvement. Most common organs involved are the gastrointestinal tract, liver, kidneys, and lungs.

Candida species form budding yeasts, hyphae, and pseudo hyphae in tissues. The pseudo hyphae can be distinguished from true hyphae by the presence of constriction at the site of septae. The tissue reaction may vary from acellular necrosis, purulent exudates, to formation of microgranulomas. Special stains like PAS and GSM stain the fungi well.

Lysis centrifugation technique has significantly improved the recovery of candidal yeast cells from blood culture. Molecular biology techniques like nucleic acid hybridization and PCR are helpful in rapid diagnosis. Both direct immunofluorescence and candidal immunohistochemistry can be performed on paraffin-embedded tissue. On electron microscopic examination, the *Candida* shows a trilaminar cell wall and fine granular cytoplasm.

Differential diagnosis of yeasts and pseudo hyphae of *Candida* includes *Cryptococcus*, *Histoplasma capsulatum*, *Blastomyces*, and *Trichosporon beigelii* (Table 4.2).

R.K. Gupta, P. Gupta (eds.), *Pathology of Opportunistic Infections*,
DOI 10.1007/978-981-10-1669-1_4

Table 4.1 Commonly encountered fungal infections in immunocompromised patients

Yeasts	Filamentous	Dimorphic
Candida	*Aspergillus*	*Histoplasma*
Cryptococcus	Zygomycetes	*Blastomyces*
Pneumocystis carinii	Phaeohyphomycosis	*Coccidioides*
Torulopsis		

From: Gupta RK. In *Pathology of opportunistic infections in tropic.* Jaypee; 2007

Table 4.2 Differentiating morphological features of common yeastlike fungi

Features	*Candida*	*Cryptococcus*	*H. capsulatum*	*Blastomyces*
Size (μm)	3–6	2–20	2–4	7–15
Shape	Spherical/oval	Pleomorphic	Spherical/oval	Spherical
No. of buds	Single/several	Single	Single	Single
Attachment of buds	Narrow	Narrow	Narrow	Very broad
Cell wall	Thin	Thin	Thin	Thick
Pseudo/true hyphae	Present	Rare	Rare	Rare
Mucicarmine stain	–	+	–	±

From: Gupta RK. In *Pathology of opportunistic infections in tropic.* Jaypee; 2007

Dermatophytosis in an Immunocompromised Patient

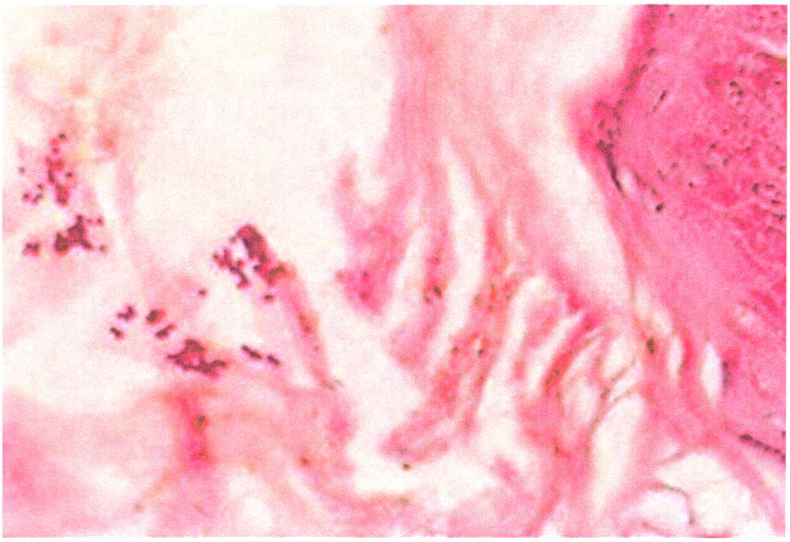

Fig. 4.1 A 28-year-old male patient known to have been on steroids for rheumatoid arthritis presented with itchy skin lesions over back for 10 days. The lesions were slightly raised with central scarring. The patient also had pallor, mild icterus, and generalized lymphadenopathy. Skin biopsy showed groups of yeastlike organisms in superficial dermis suggestive of dermatophytosis (PAS ×400)

Candidiasis in a Patient of CIS Buccal Mucosa

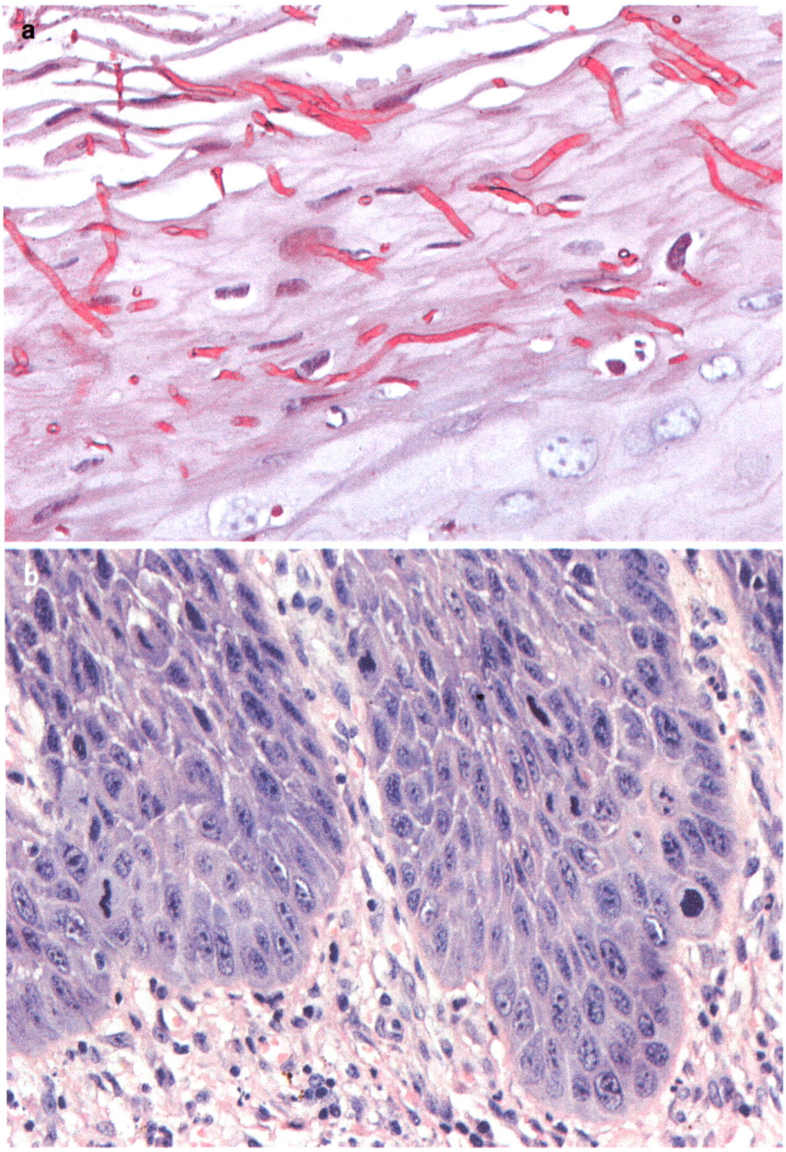

Fig. 4.2 (**a**, **b**) A 48-year-old female patient with prolonged h/o tobacco chewing presented with an ulcerated growth on the mucosa of the left cheek. The lesion was about 3 × 2 cm in size. Cervical lymph nodes were not enlarged. Chest X-ray and laboratory workup were WNL. The biopsy from the ulcer showed pseudo hyphae and yeasts of *Candida* (**a** PAS ×400) along with CIS (**b** HE ×200)

Candidiasis in a Patient of Keratinizing Squamous Cell Carcinoma Tongue

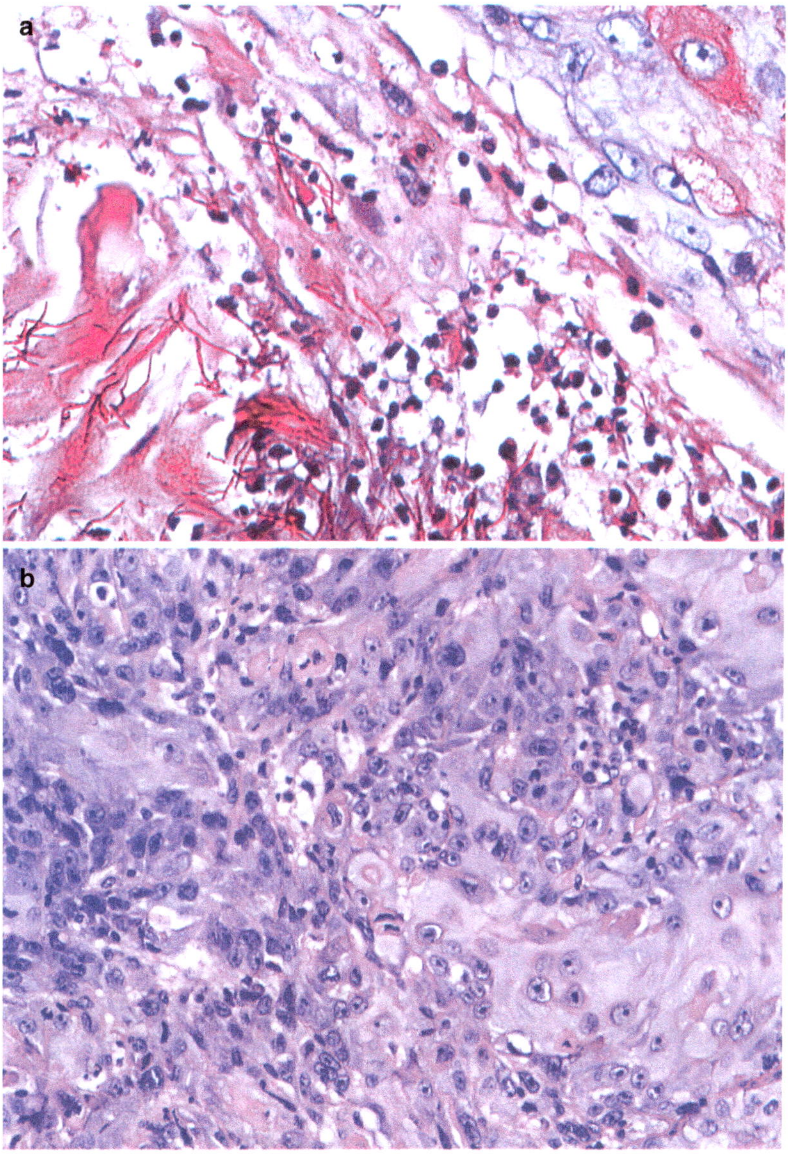

Fig. 4.3 (**a**, **b**) A 36-year-old male patient with h/o tobacco chewing for >20 years presented with ulcerated swelling measuring 3 × 2 cm on the right lateral margin of the tongue. Lymph nodes in the drainage area were not involved. Punch biopsy from the lesion showed plenty of hyphae and pseudo hyphae of *Candida* (**a** PAS ×400) along with keratinizing squamous cell carcinoma (**b** HE ×200)

Candidiasis in a Patient of Keratinizing Squamous Cell Carcinoma Esophagus

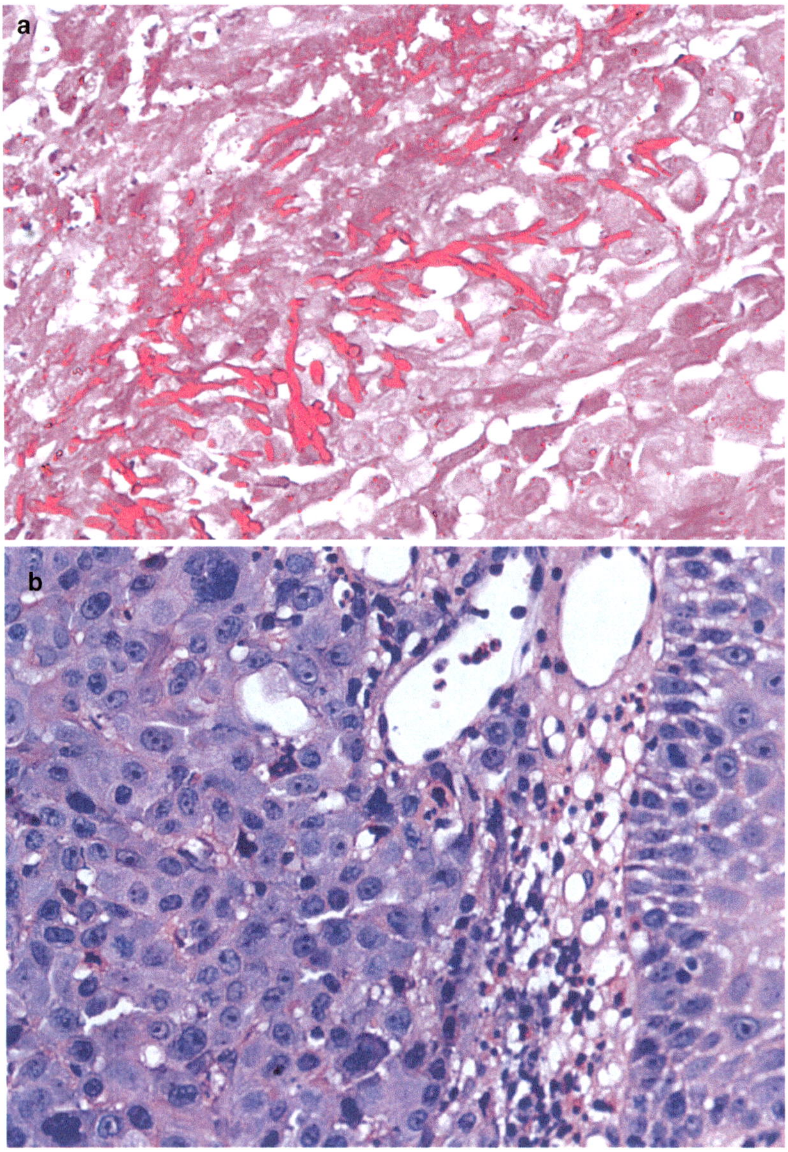

Fig. 4.4 (**a**, **b**) A 50-year-old female patient presented with progressively increasing dysphagia. Upper GI endoscopy showed an ulceroproliferative friable growth in lower 1/3 of esophageal region. Endoscopic esophageal biopsy from the growth showed budding yeasts and pseudo hyphae of *Candida* (**a** PAS ×400) along with keratinizing squamous cell carcinoma of esophagus (**b** HE ×200)

Candidiasis in a Patient of Nonkeratinizing Squamous Cell Carcinoma Esophagus

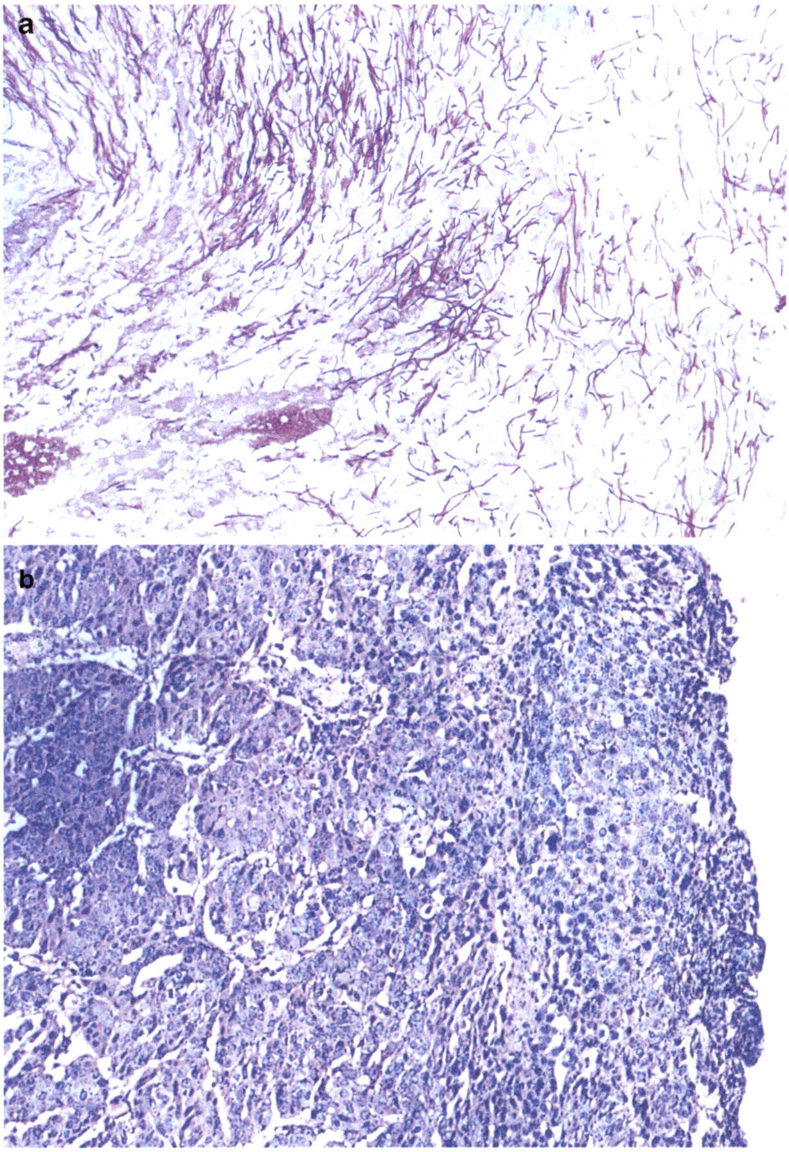

Fig. 4.5 (**a**, **b**) A 45-year-old female patient presented with progressively increasing dysphagia (grade III). Upper GI endoscopy showed a friable growth in mid esophageal region. Endoscopic esophageal biopsy from the growth showed pseudo hyphae, hyphae, and a few budding yeasts of *Candida* (**a** PAS ×200) along with non-keratinizing squamous cell carcinoma (**b** HE ×100)

Candidiasis in a Patient of Undifferentiated Carcinoma Esophagus

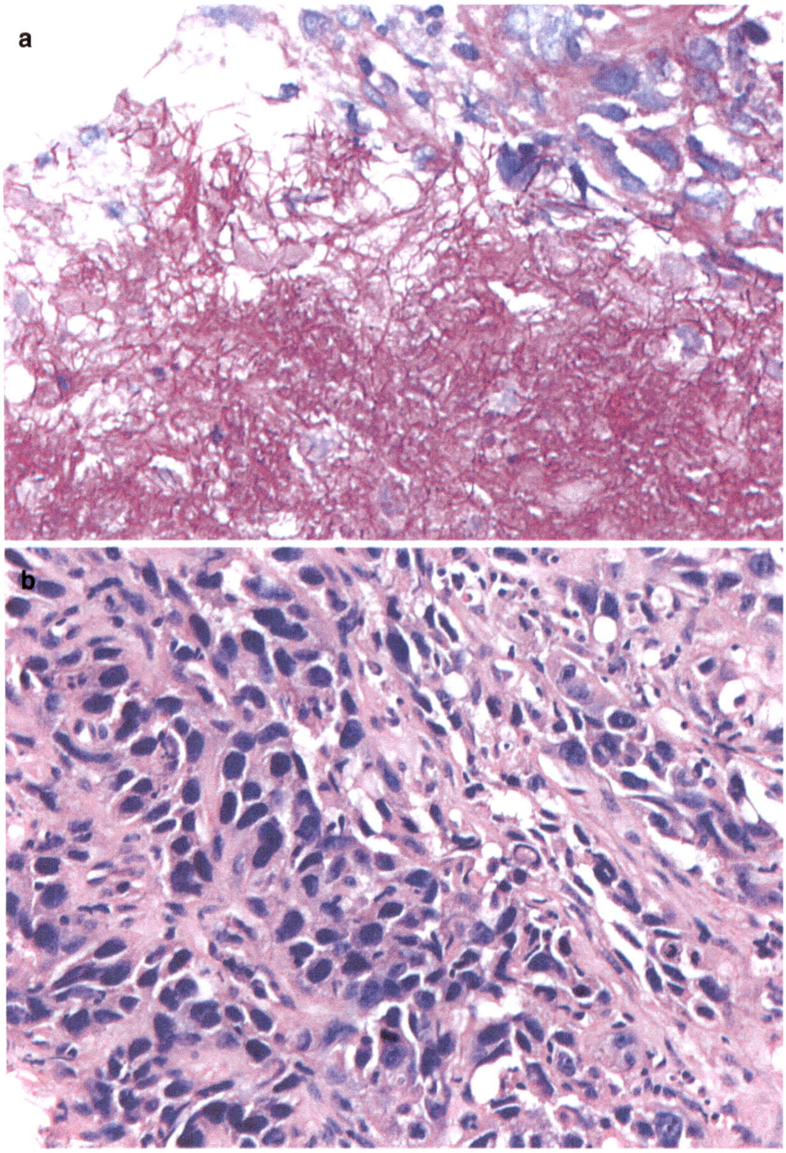

Fig. 4.6 (**a**, **b**) A 74-year-old male patient presented with dysphagia and odynophagia for 6 weeks followed by weakness. Upper GI endoscopy revealed an ulcerated mid esophageal growth; endoscopic biopsy was obtained. Histological examination revealed the presence of plenty of pseudo hyphae of *Candida* (**a** PAS ×400) along with undifferentiated carcinoma esophagus (**b** HE ×200)

Candidiasis in a Patient of Adenocarcinoma GE Junction

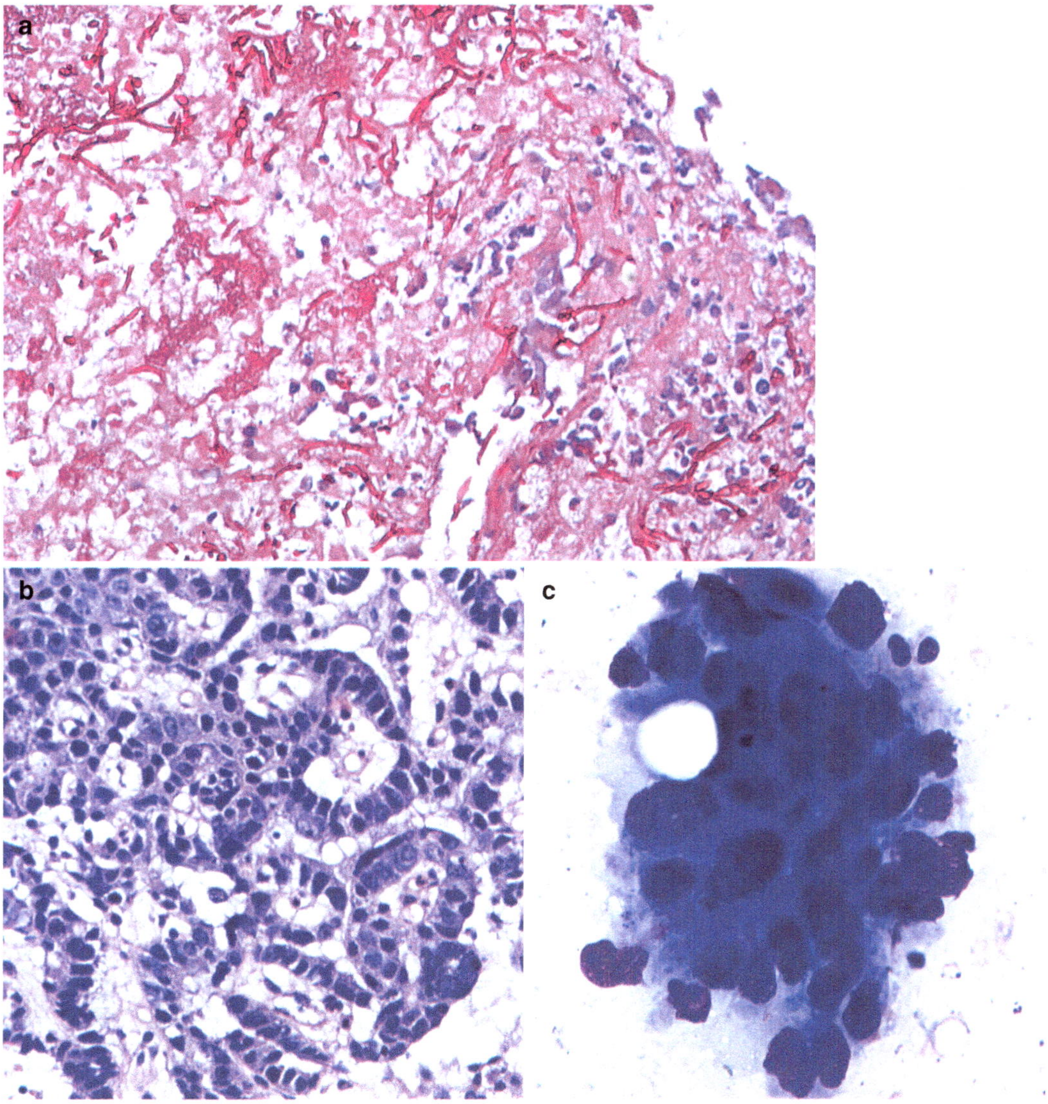

Fig. 4.7 (**a**–**c**) A 38-year-old female patient presented with abdominal pain and melena. Ultrasonography of the upper abdomen revealed enlarged liver showing fatty change and multiple necrotic SOL with portal vein thrombosis and enlarged peripancreatic lymph nodes. Upper GI endoscopy revealed a polypoidal growth at GE junction. The biopsy from the polyp showed hyphae, pseudo hyphae, and budding yeasts of *Candida* (**a** PAS ×400) along with adenocarcinoma of GE junction (**b** HE ×200); guided FNAC of the liver nodule showed metastatic adenocarcinoma (**c** MGG ×400)

Candidiasis Stomach in a Patient of Adenocarcinoma Stomach

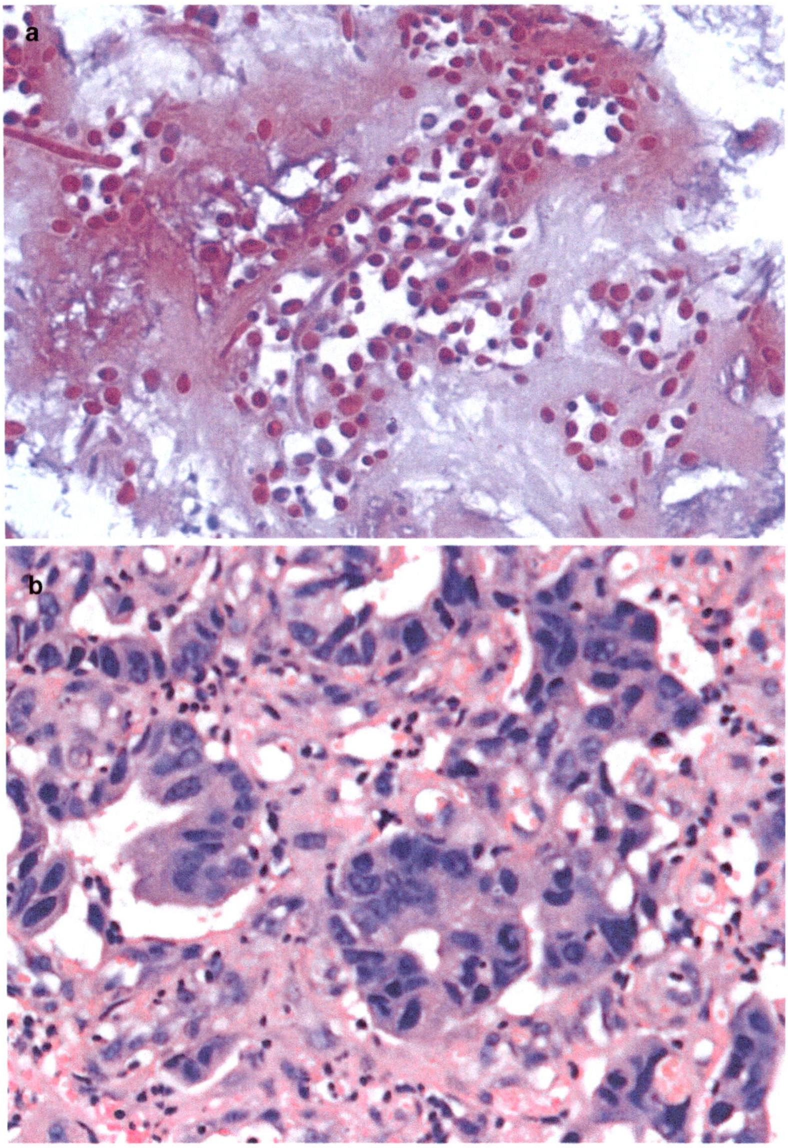

Fig. 4.8 (**a**, **b**) A 55-year-old male patient presented with melena. Upper GI endoscopy revealed an ulcerated gastric central polyp. The biopsy from the polyp showed hyphae, pseudo hyphae, and budding yeasts of *Candida* (**a** PAS ×400) along with adenocarcinoma of the stomach (**b** HE ×200)

Candidiasis in a Case of Poorly Differentiated Adenocarcinoma of the Ampula

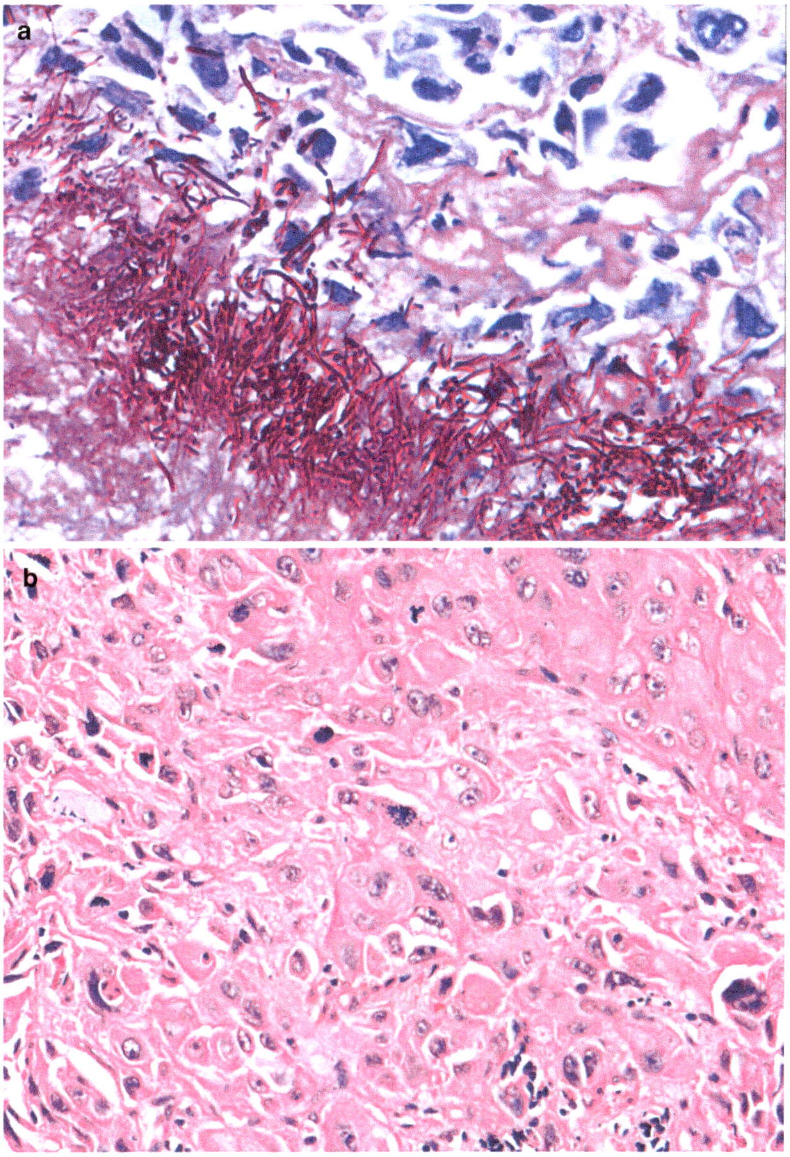

Fig. 4.9 (**a**, **b**) A 55-year-old male patient presented with itching, anorexia, weakness, and jaundice for 1 month. USG showed dilated CBD with block at papilla. Upper GI endoscopy revealed an ulcerated mass at papilla and a biopsy was obtained. Histological examination revealed the presence of yeastlike bodies and plenty of pseudo hyphae of *Candida* (**a** PAS ×400) along with poorly differentiated adenocarcinoma of the ampula (**b** HE ×200)

Candidiasis in Bronchial Cast in an Immunocompromised Patient

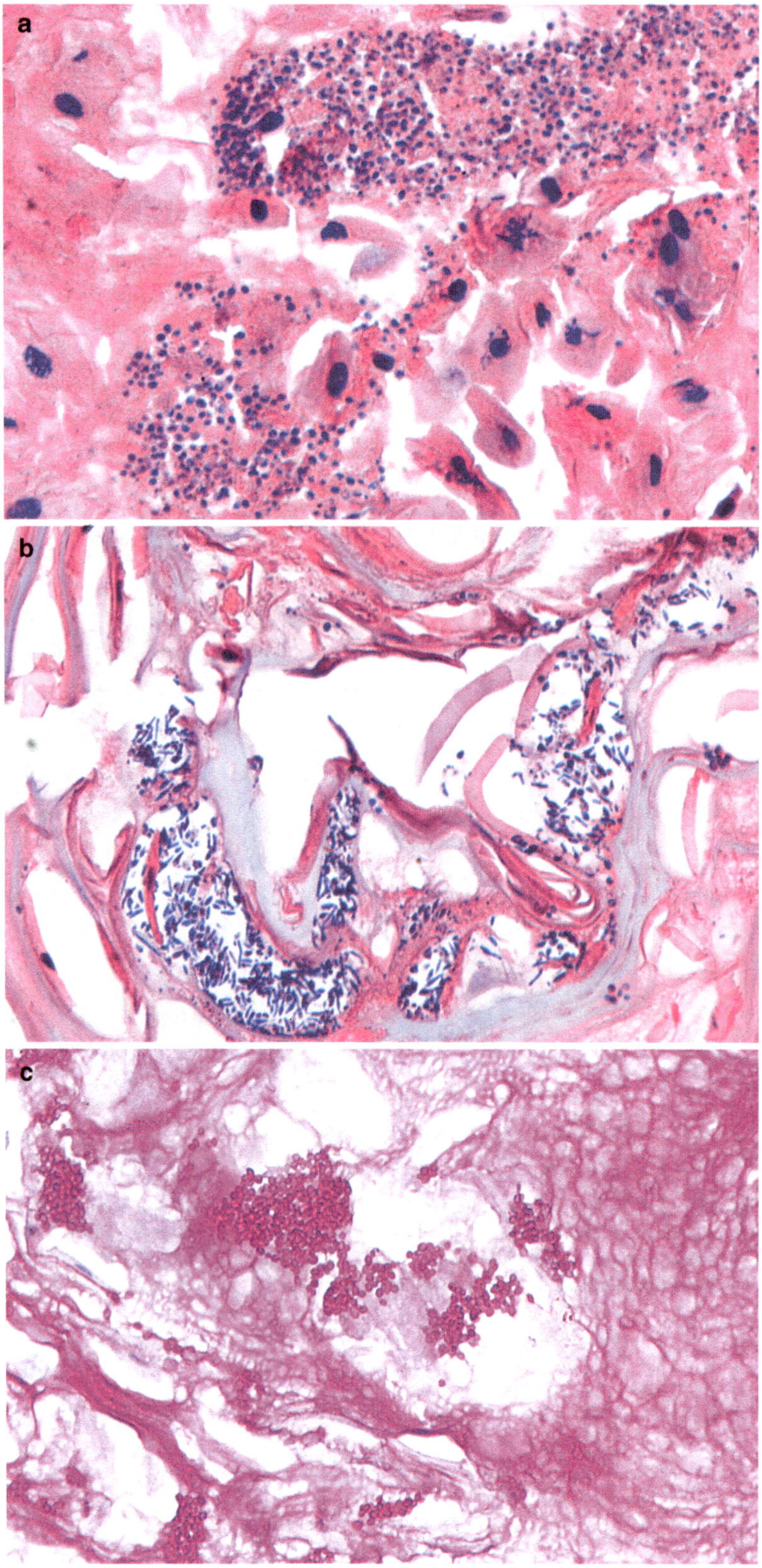

Fig. 4.10 (**a**–**c**) A 47-year-old female patient developed postcholecystectomy cholangitis with fever, septicemia, and acute renal failure for which she received 20 sittings of hemodialysis; however, her clinical condition continued to deteriorate and she passed into coma. Blood counts revealed polymorphonuclear leukocytosis with total WBC count of 15,300/cu mm with 75 % neutrophils; patient had thrombocytopenia with platelet count of 46,000/cu mm. Her serum creatinine was 4.0 mg/dl and serum urea was 56.2 mg/dl. She continued to receive hemodialysis. During endotracheal suction, a necrotic soft tissue piece was sucked out. On histopathological examination, it revealed necrotic tissue with some degenerated squamous cells and plenty of budding yeasts and pseudo hyphae of *Candida* (**a**, **b** HE ×400, **c** PAS ×400)

Candidiasis Lung in a Renal Allograft Recipient

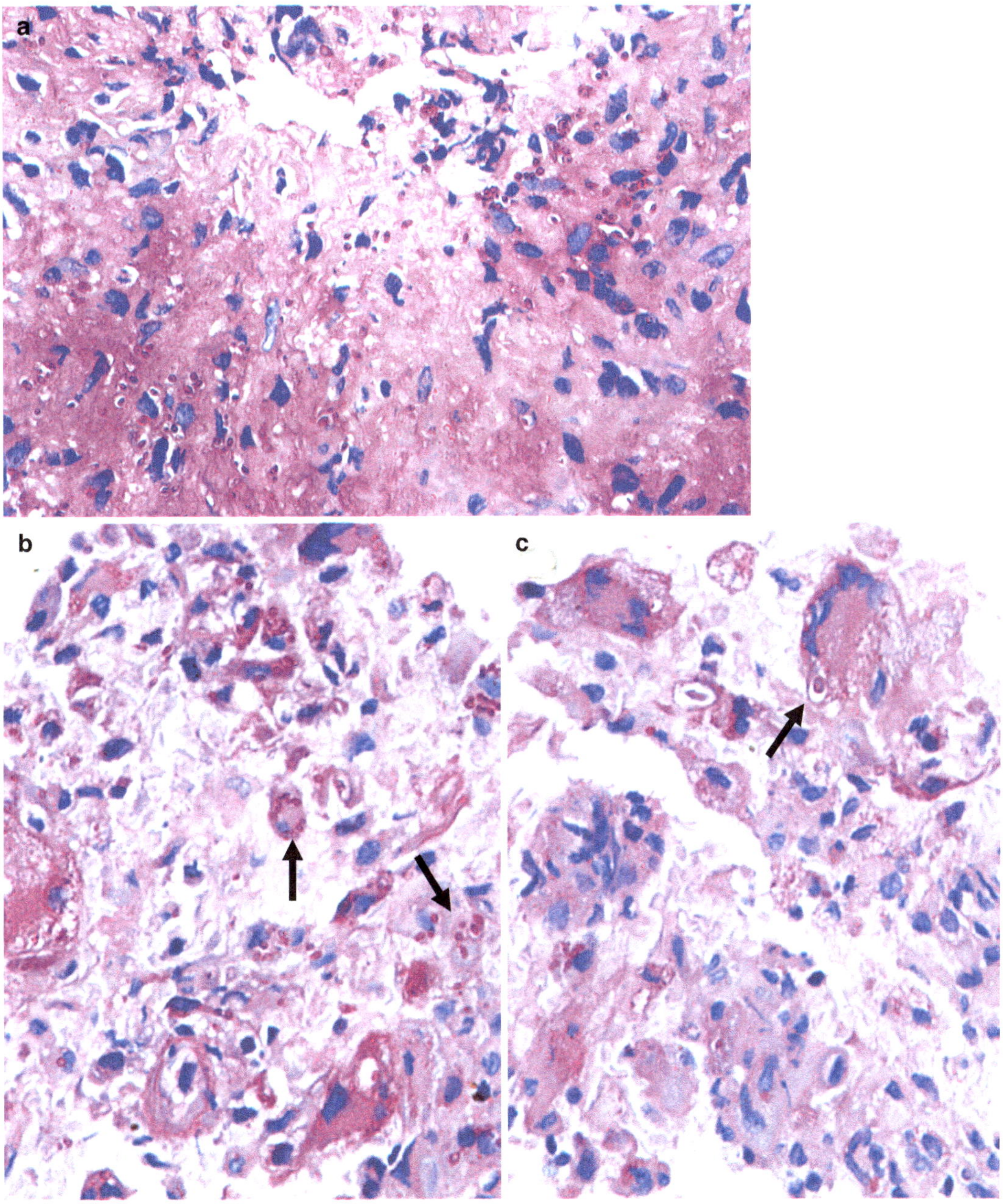

Fig. 4.11 (**a**–**d**) A 30-year-old male patient receiving live-related renal allograft was being maintained on triple drug immunosuppression. Six weeks posttransplant, he presented with acute graft dysfunction with rise in serum creatinine. Routine chest X-ray (PA) revealed nodular consolidation; CT-guided needle core biopsy from the nodule was performed. The histopathological examination revealed multiple ill-defined collections of epithelioid cells, macrophages, and few giant cells along with plentiful budding yeastlike fungus with occasional pseudo hyphae, the fungus was present both within the macrophages and giant cells (*arrows*) as well as extracellularly (**a**–**c** PAS ×400, **d** CSM ×400)

Fig. 4.11 (continued)

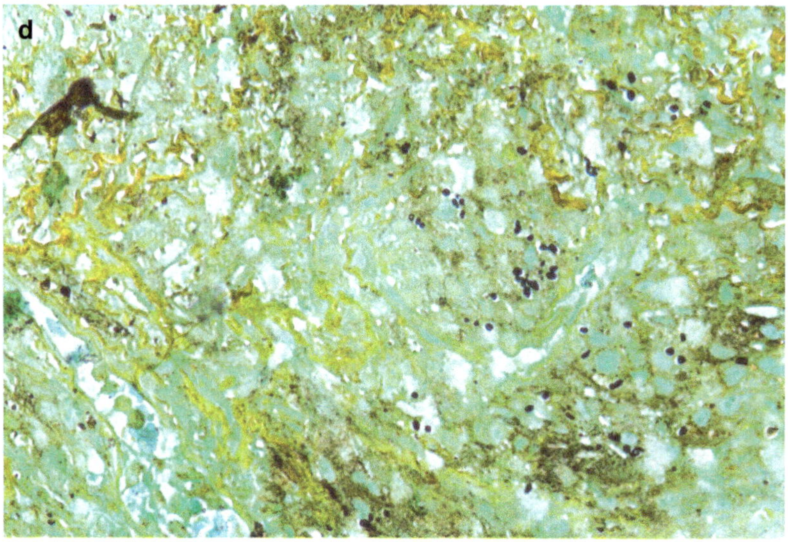

Candidiasis Kidney in a Patient of ALL

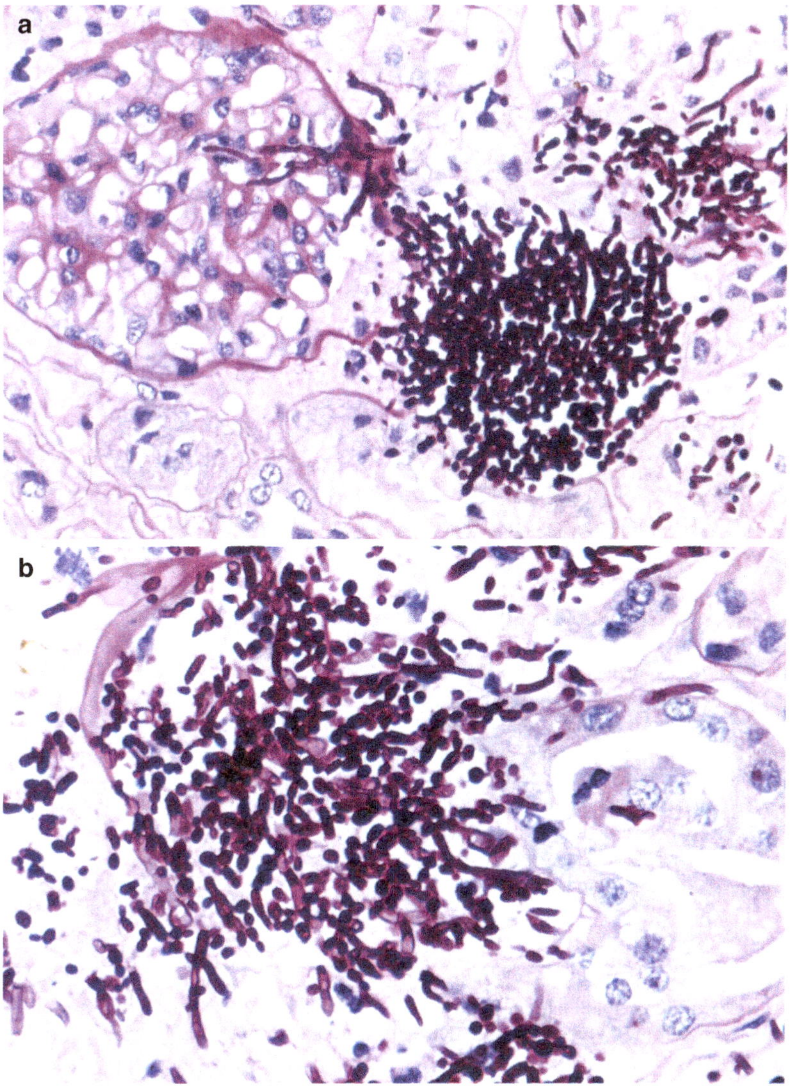

Fig. 4.12 (**a**, **b**) A 30-year-old male patient known to have been suffering from ALL was admitted to the hospital with fever, generalized body ache, progressively increasing jaundice, and tenderness in both loins. Ultrasonographic examination of the abdomen revealed mild hepatomegaly and multiple enlarged retroperitoneal lymph nodes; both kidneys were of normal size. Laboratory workup revealed that the patient had severe anemia with hemoglobin level of 3.6 g/dl; total WBC count was 36,600/cu mm with 82% lymphoblasts in peripheral circulation, and the platelet count was 52,000/cu mm. Serum bilirubin was 16.8 mg/dl (direct 8.9 mg/dl and indirect 7.9 mg/dl), SGPT was 63 IU/dl, and SGOT was 54 IU/dl. Blood culture did not grow any organisms up to 72 h. The patient died 4th day after hospitalization. Postmortem renal biopsy showed budding yeasts and pseudo hyphae of Candida infiltrating renal parenchyma (**a**, **b** PAS ×400) (From: Gupta RK. In *Pathology of opportunistic infections in tropic*. Jaypee; 2007)

Candidiasis Renal Pelvis in a Diabetic Patient

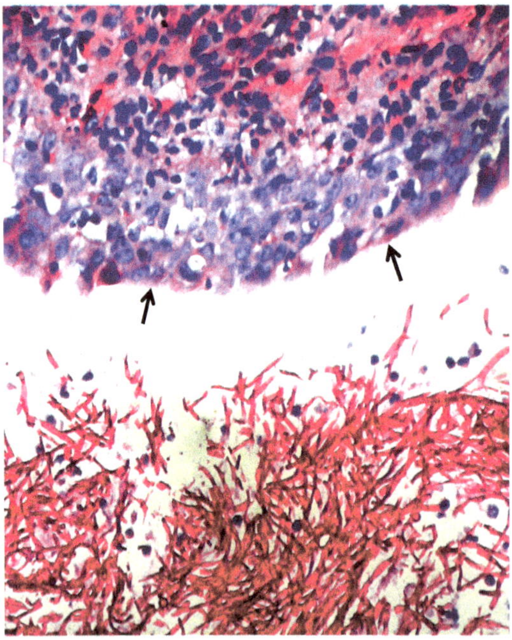

Fig. 4.13 A 54-year-old female patient, who had been suffering with diabetic glomerulosclerosis, received live-related renal allograft. Three years posttransplant, she presented with progressive graft dysfunction and anemia. Graft biopsy was inconclusive. While in the hospital, she passed grayish white fragments in the urine. Histopathological examination of these fragments revealed the structure of renal papilla (*arrows*) along with pseudo hyphae and yeastlike organisms suggestive of candidiasis of the renal pelvis (PAS ×400)

Fig. 4.14 (**a**–**d**) A39-year-old female patient known to have been suffering with chronic kidney disease (CKD) and chronic lung disease (CLD) presented with h/o low backache for 1 year along with lower abdominal pain which increased in severity with inspiration followed by fever, nausea, loss of appetite, and loss of weight. Laboratory workup revealed that the patient was moderately anemic with hemoglobin level of 7.0 g/dl and total WBC count was 13,900/cu mm with 78 % polys. Her serum creatinine was 3.1 mg/dl. USG of the abdomen revealed that both kidneys were small, and a subcapsular mid polar mass was also identified in the right kidney. Clinical diagnosis of subcapsular hematoma of the right kidney was considered. Right PCN drained small amount of altered blood which was sterile on culture. PCD was removed after 4 days. During postoperative period, the patient received broad-spectrum antibiotics; postoperative recovery was uneventful, and the patient was discharged on the 10th day after hospitalization. Four months later, she again presented with fever and left ventricular failure. 2-D echo showed rounded 27 × 20 mm mass in anterior papillary muscle of the left ventricle. At surgery anterior leaflet of the mitral valve was found prolapsed with torn out chordae. Anterior leaflet of the mitral valve along with anterior papillary muscle of the left ventricle was excised. The postoperative recovery was uneventful. Gross examination of the resected specimen revealed anterior leaflet of mitral valve measuring 3.0 cm along with a globular soft tissue piece (papillary muscle) measuring 2 cm, its cut surface showed brownish yellow areas (**a**). Histological examination of the mitral valve leaflet revealed myxoid change with areas of geographical necrosis and that of the papillary muscle revealed necrotic area with microabscess formation infiltrated with mixed inflammatory infiltrate, histiocytes, and giant cells (**b** HE ×200) along with plentiful budding yeastlike fungus with the presence of pseudo hyphae (**c** PAS ×400, **d** CSM ×400). Diagnosis of candidiasis of the anterior papillary muscle of the left ventricle was offered

Candidiasis of Papillary Muscle of the Left Ventricle of the Heart in an Immunocompromised Patient (Chronic Kidney Disease)

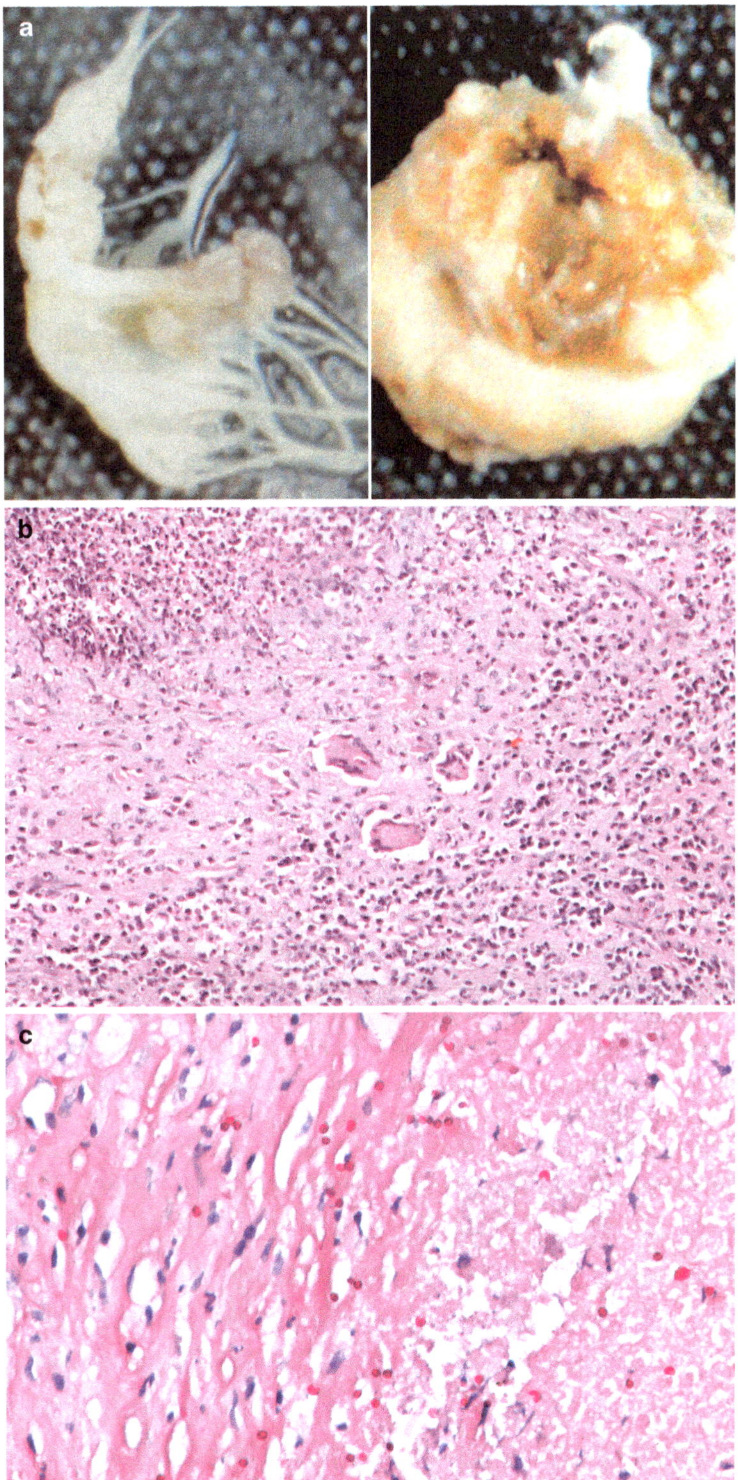

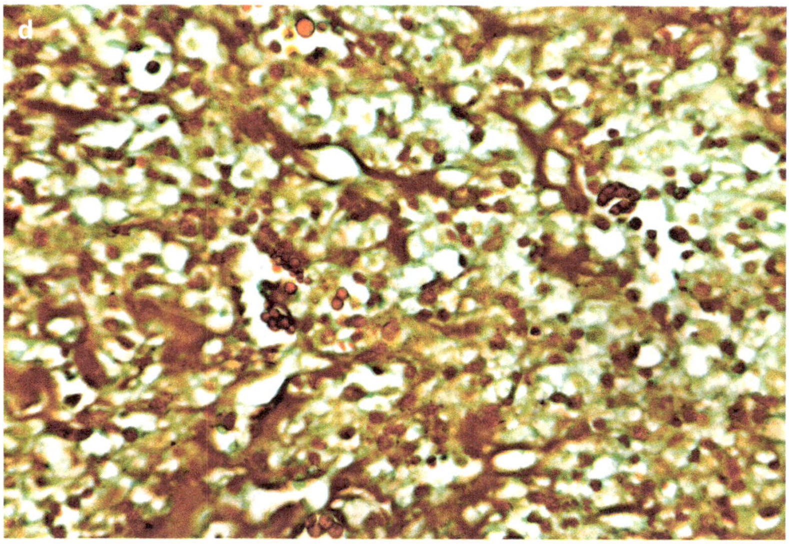

Fig. 4.14 (continued)

Cryptococcus **(Syn. Torulosis, European Blastomycosis):** Among various species of the genus *Cryptococcus*, *Cryptococcus neoformans* is the only human pathogen. *C. neoformans* is a 3.5–8 μm budding yeast; the budding is single with a narrow neck between the daughter and the parent cells. The fungal elements are surrounded by a mucopolysaccharide capsule which appears as a halo around the cell.

C. neoformans is a natural habitant of soil, particularly the soil mixed with excreta of turkeys, pigeons, starlings, and other birds. The fungus is acquired by inhalation of contaminated dust into the lungs. Conditions associated with defective cellular immunity such as HIV/AIDS, long-term corticosteroid therapy, chemotherapeutic immunosuppressive agents, diabetes mellitus, solid organ transplants, and hematopoietic and lymphoreticular malignancies predispose the patients to cryptococcosis.

Two major sites of involvement are the lungs and cerebro-meninges. The fungus is extremely neurotropic with fulminant course. Disseminated infection involving the skin, bone and joints, and kidneys may also occur.

Definitive diagnosis of *C. neoformans* can be made by demonstration of fungal yeasts on India ink preparation in CSF and by culture. Latex agglutination test can be used for the demonstration of cryptococcal antigen in CSF. Riu stain may be used to demonstrate cryptococci in smears prepared from bronchial brushings and needle aspirates.

Histological examination of the tissue specimen often shows acellular necrosis and heavily encapsulated yeast cells. Direct fluorescent techniques may help in the diagnosis of chronic cryptococcal lesions. On electron microscopic examination, the capsule shows a finely granular matrix with radiating filaments and tubules.

Cryptococcal Meningitis in an Immunocompromised Patient (Long-Standing Pulmonary Tuberculosis)

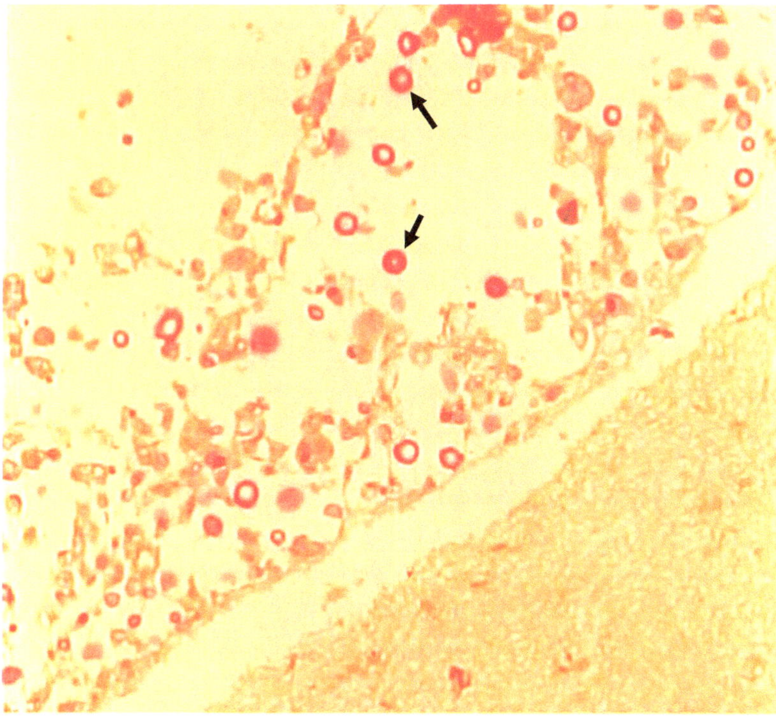

Fig. 4.15 A 35-year-old male patient who had been suffering from long-standing pulmonary tuberculosis and was on irregular antitubercular treatment, presented with low-grade fever with evening rise of temperature, headache, and diminution of vision for 1 month. The clinical examination revealed that the patient was in altered state of sensorium, responding only to painful stimuli with bilateral papilledema and VI and VII cranial nerve paresis. Chest X-ray revealed pleural thickening. Cranial CT showed a ring lesion in the right parietal region. CSF examination revealed protein 40 mg/dl and sugar 50 mg/dl; there was no pleocytosis. Serum and CSF were negative for antimycobacterial antibody but were positive for cryptococcal antigen. India ink preparation showed budding forms of cryptococci and *Cryptococcus neoformans* was isolated on CSF culture. The patient received amphotericin and anti-edema measures but succumbed to his illness the next day. At autopsy the meninges were hazy and histological examination revealed plenty of cryptococci in meningeal space suggestive of cryptococcal meningitis (Masson-Fontana ×400) (Contributors – Dr. Anita Mahadevan and Prof. SK Shankar, Human Brain Bank, Department of Neuropathology, NIMHANS, Bangalore, India) (From: Gupta RK. In *Pathology of opportunistic infections in tropic*. Jaypee; 2007)

Cryptococcal Meningitis in a Patient of Idiopathic CD4 Lymphocytopenia

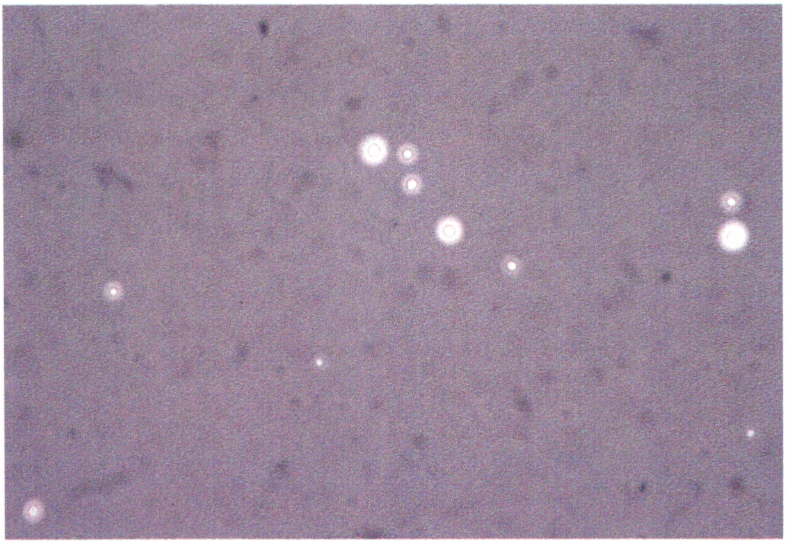

Fig. 4.16 A 50-year-old male patient presented with mild to moderate fever without any localizing symptoms for 8 months and abnormal movements of the right upper limb for 2 weeks. Two weeks earlier, he developed holocranial headache associated with "paroxysmal tremor"-like movements both at rest and activity but not during sleep. He also had inability to hold objects in the right hand. He had lost 8 kg of weight during the past 8 months. Fever did not respond to various antibiotics and antitubercular therapy. Clinical examination, except for the presence of coarse tremors, was WNL. Laboratory investigations revealed TLC of 6600/cu mm with 20 % lymphocytes (absolute lymphocyte count of 1320/cu mm). Bone marrow examination did not reveal any abnormality. The patient was nondiabetic, and other laboratory parameters including liver and renal function tests were WNL. Chest X-ray did not reveal any abnormality. Multiple blood and urine culture were negative for tuberculosis, fungus, and pyogenic organisms. US of the abdomen did not reveal any organomegaly, and 2D echocardiography was normal. MRI of the brain showed a large lesion in the frontoparietal and right occipital region, which was hypertense in T2-weighted images. CSF examination showed mildly elevated proteins (80 mg/dl) with lymphocytic pleocytosis, India ink preparation showed capsulated yeasts of cryptococci. CSF was also positive for cryptococcal antigen by latex agglutination and was negative for IgM anti-toxoplasma antibody. Serology for CMV and HIV-1 and HIV-2 was negative. CD4 cell count was 17/μl. Patient responded well to the therapy (Courtesy Neurology India. Photograph courtesy Prof. KN Prasad, Department of Microbiology, Sanjay Gandhi Postgraduate Institute of Medical Sciences, Lucknow, India) (From: Gupta RK. In *Pathology of opportunistic infections in tropic*. Jaypee; 2007)

Cryptococcosis-FNAC from Lung Mass in an HIV-Positive Patient

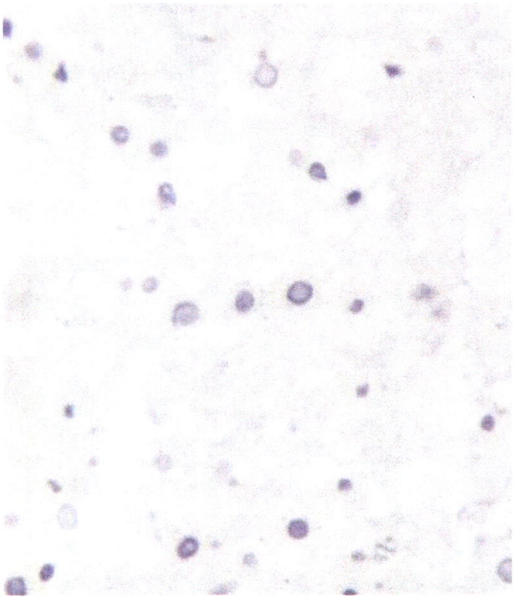

Fig. 4.17 A 25-year-old female patient presented with cough and breathlessness for 1 month. She was found to be HIV positive. Chest X-ray revealed mass in the upper lobe of the right lung with erosion of the overlying rib. CT-guided aspiration of the mass showed capsulated budding yeastlike bodies suggestive of *Cryptococcus* (Melanin ×400) (Contributor – Dr. S Radha, Aware Global Hospital, Hyderabad, India)

Cryptococcosis of the Kidney in a Renal Allograft Recipient

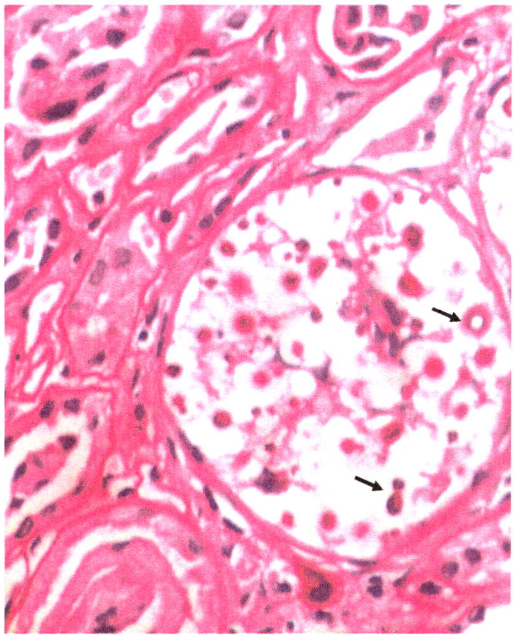

Fig. 4.18 A 37-year-old male renal allograft recipient who was HBsAg positive, 1 year posttransplant, presented with rising serum creatinine, proteinuria, and deteriorating liver functions. The patient was suspected to have chronic transplant nephropathy with chronic liver disease. During hospital stay, the patient developed hepatic encephalopathy and died. Postmortem kidney biopsy revealed tubules filled with capsulated, spherical budding yeastlike organisms surrounded by a clear halo suggestive of cryptococcosis (PAS ×400) (From: Gupta RK. In *Pathology of opportunistic infections in tropic*. Jaypee; 2007)

Cryptococcosis of the Lung in a Patient of Wagner's Granulomatosis

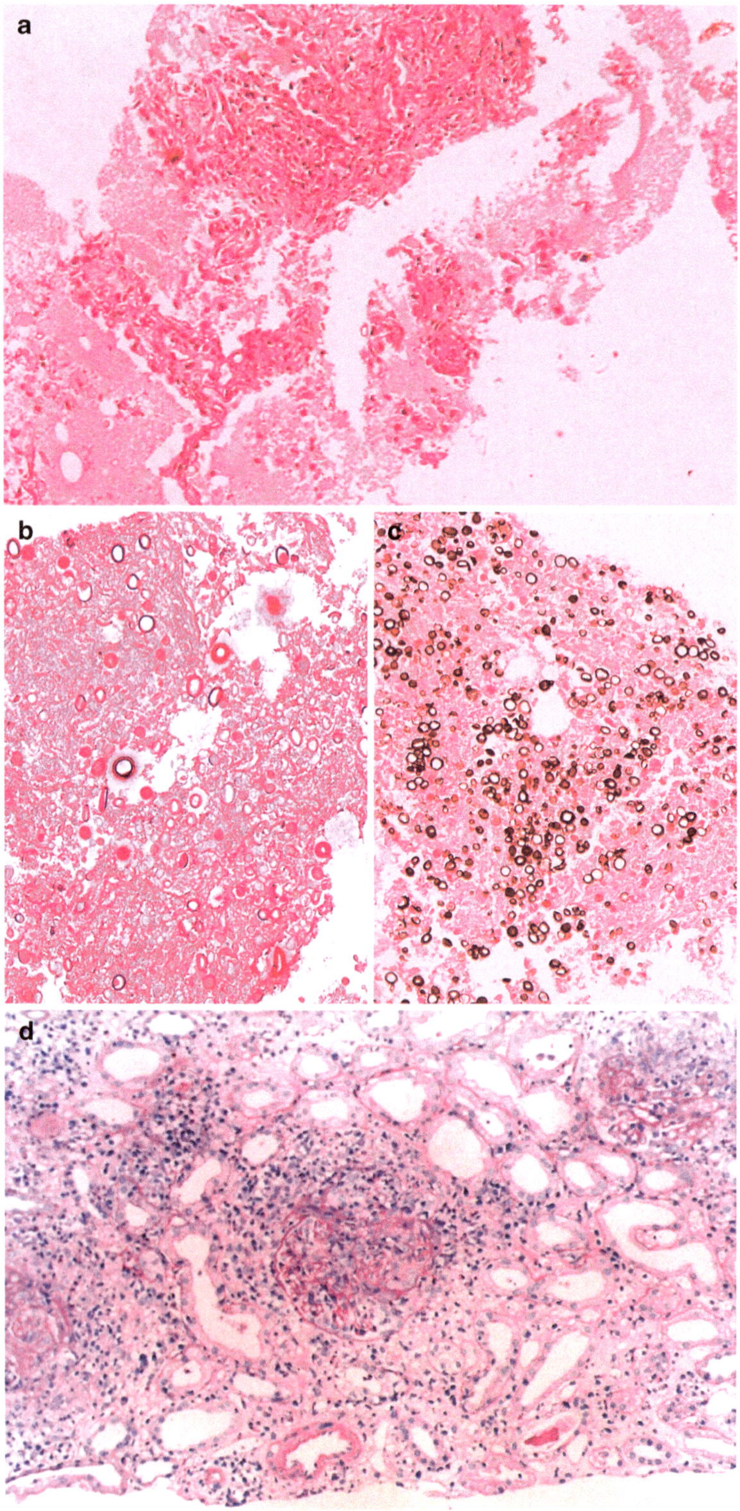

Fig. 4.19 (**a**–**d**) A 57-year-old male patient known to have pauci-immune crescentic glomerulonephritis on steroid and cyclophosphamide presented with fever, decreased appetite, and weight loss (11 kg) since 4 months. The patient was empirically on ATT before presentation to the hospital. He had no lymphadenopathy. Routine hematological workup revealed hemoglobin 11.5 g/dl, and total WBC count was 5600/cu mm, with N-59, L-38, E-1, and M-2 %, respectively; ESR was 16 mm. The patient was nondiabetic; he tested negative for HBsAg, HCV, and HIV. Further laboratory workup revealed C-ANCA 40 U/ml, HbA1c 5.7 %, and serum ACE 23 U/l. Sputum smear was negative for AFB; sputum culture was also negative for tubercle bacilli. Chest CT showed a nodular lesion with eccentric cavitation in the upper lobe of the right lung, and small nodular lesions in the upper lobe of the left lung were also identified; mediastinal lymph nodes were enlarged. CT-guided biopsy from the right upper lobe of the lung showed noncaseating epithelioid granuloma (**a**. HE ×200); Ziehl-Neelsen stain for AFB was negative. The lung biopsy also showed plenty of capsulated, spherical budding yeastlike organisms surrounded by a clear halo suggestive of cryptococcosis (**b** HE ×400 and **c** PAS ×400). The renal biopsy revealed necrotizing crescentric glomerulonephritis (**d** PAS ×200)

Cryptococcosis of the Sternoclavicular Joint in a Diabetic Patient

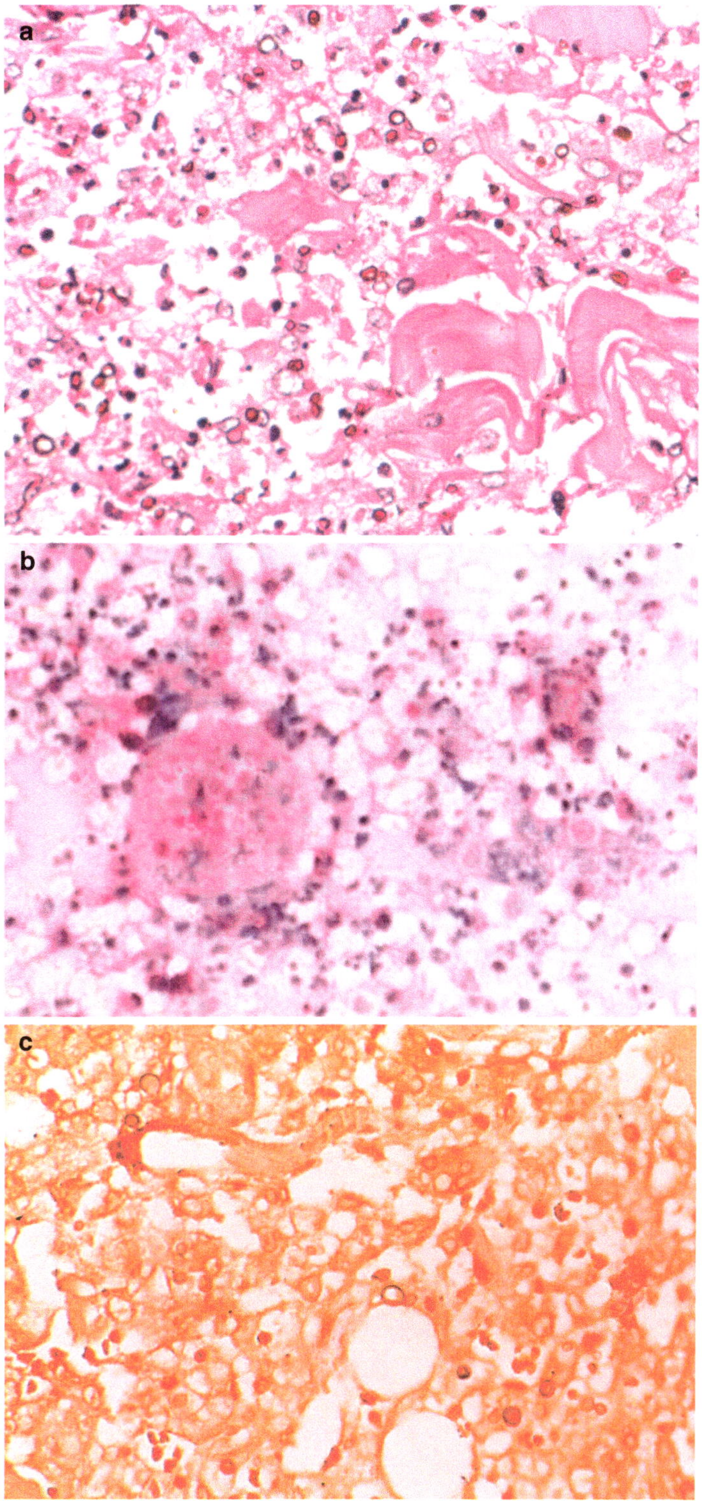

Fig. 4.20 (**a**–**c**) A 60-year-old male diabetic patient presented with fever, anemia, drowsiness, gastrointestinal bleeds, and mental confusion. Radiological evaluation revealed multiple skeletal hypodense areas which on FNAC revealed mixed inflammatory infiltrate with few giant cells and capsulated yeastlike bodies both extracellular and intracellular within the histiocytes and giant cells, suggestive of cryptococcosis (**a** HE ×400, **b** PAS ×400 and **c** Masson-Fontana ×400) (From: Gupta RK. In *Pathology of opportunistic infections in tropic*. Jaypee; 2007)

Pneumocystis carinii: *Pneumocystis carinii* is a nonfilamentous fungus. Three developmental stages, viz., trophozoites, precysts (5–8 μm), and the cysts of *P. carinii*, are recognized. Trophozoites are infective. The infection is possibly acquired through human contact via inhalation of infected droplets and leads to the development of pneumonia. The organisms remain extracellular. *Pneumocystis carinii pneumonia* (PCP) is one of the leading opportunistic infection and the major cause of morbidity and mortality in patients of HIV/AIDS. HIV-infected patients with CD4 counts <200 cells/cu mm are at higher risk of contracting PCP. Other predisposing conditions include solid organ transplantation, prolonged immunosuppressive therapy, leukemias, and other hematological malignancies.

These patients often present as pneumonia with fever and respiratory symptoms. The disease is rapidly progressive and associated with high morbidity and mortality unless diagnosed and treated promptly. At autopsy extrapulmonary lesions involving the lymph nodes, bone marrow, spleen, liver, adrenals, and GIT have been documented in 1–3 % of these cases. Cotrimoxazole affords effective chemoprophylaxis.

Histopathological examination of the lung biopsy shows cohesive granular alveolar exudates with foamy honeycomb appearance which appears eosinophilic on HE stain. The foamy material is composed of aggregates of trophozoites with intermingled cyst forms. The cyst forms are stained pink with PAS and black with GSM satins. The organisms appear as boat-shaped or helmet-shaped bodies on cytological evaluation of bronchoalveolar lavage. On electron microscopy, characteristic segmentally thickened double membrane of the cyst wall is seen.

Differential diagnosis includes other yeastlike fungi such as *C. albicans, C. neoformans,* and *H. capsulatum.*

Pneumocystis Carinii Pneumonia in a Renal Allograft Recipient

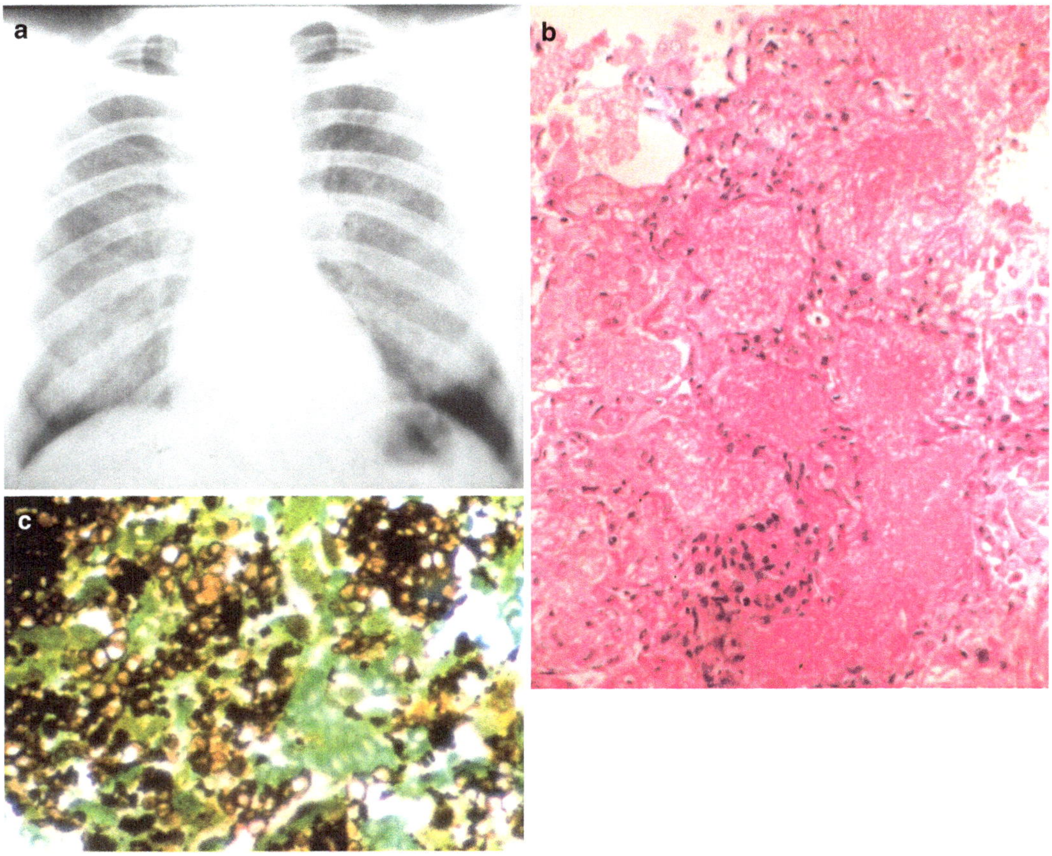

Fig. 4.21 (**a**–**c**) A 36-year-old male patient who received live-related renal allograft, 3-month posttransplant presented with fever and chills along with cough and breathlessness of short duration. Chest X-ray (PA view) showed extensive bilateral patchy consolidation (**a**). The patient died 3 days after hospitalization. Postmortem lung biopsy revealed foamy acellular PAS-positive alveolar exudates (**b**. PAS ×400); on CSM stain, the exudate showed multiple rounded or oval organisms suggestive of *Pneumocystis carinii* (**c**. CSM ×400) (From: Gupta RK. In *Pathology of opportunistic infections in tropic*. Jaypee; 2007)

Pneumocystis carinii Pneumonia in a Renal Allograft Recipient

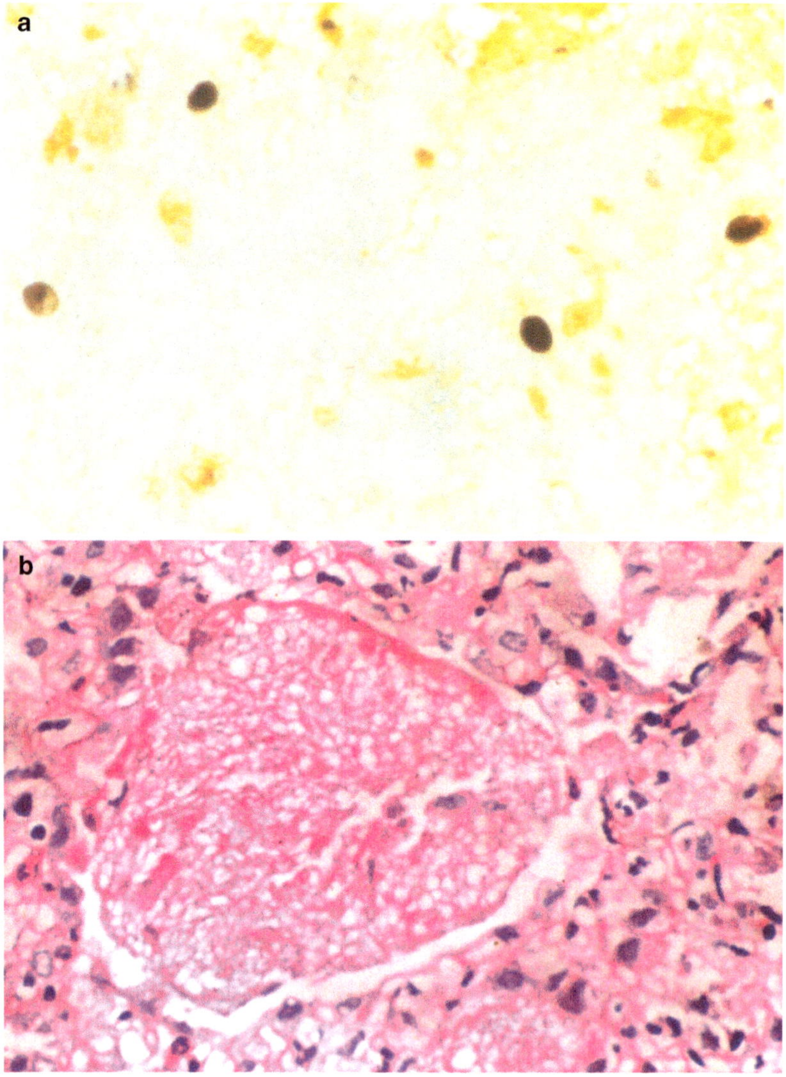

Fig. 4.22 (**a**, **b**) An 18-year-old male patient received live-related renal allograft 6 years back. He presented with irregular fever for 4 months and dry cough and breathlessness for 10 days. Chest X-ray showed left lung consolidation. Bronchoalveolar lavage showed boat-shaped cysts of *P. carinii* (**a** CSM ×400). Transbronchial lung biopsy revealed foamy acellular PAS-positive alveolar exudates suggestive of *P. carinii* (**b** PAS ×400). The patient responded to cotrimoxazole and recovered (From: Gupta RK. In *Pathology of opportunistic infections in tropic*. Jaypee; 2007)

Torulopsis glabrata **(Causative Agent of Torulopsosis):** *Torulopsis glabrata* is a rare opportunistic fungal pathogen. In immunocompromised host, it usually presents as urinary tract infection. It does not produce hyphae or pseudo hyphae on culture.

In tissue, it forms small yeast cells which are extracellular and appear in irregular aggregates. Tissue reaction may be minimal. However, at times, microabscesses may be recognized. Definitive diagnosis can be established by direct immunofluorescence on paraffin-embedded tissue.

Torulopsis in Urine Culture of a Renal Allograft Recipient

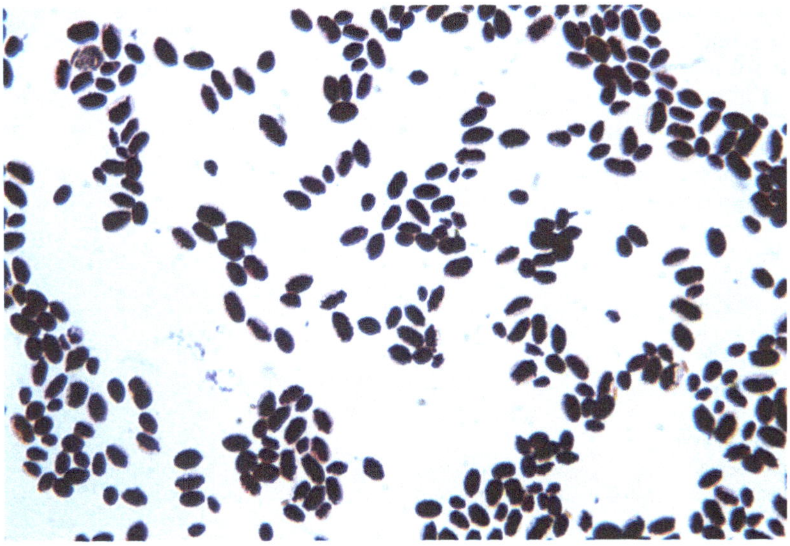

Fig. 4.23 Smear from urine culture of a renal allograft recipient showing Gram-positive yeast forms of *Torulopsis* (Grams stain ×1000) (Contributor – Prof. K N Prasad, Department of Microbiology, Sanjay Gandhi Postgraduate Institute of Medical Sciences, Lucknow, Inida) (From: Gupta RK. In *Pathology of opportunistic infections in tropic*. Jaypee; 2007)

Aspergillus **Species (Causative Agent of Aspergillosis):** *Aspergillus* infection is acquired by inhalation or direct contact with contaminated dust. The infection may also be iatrogenic through contaminated surgical instruments, intraocular lens, prosthetic devices, and catheters. Aspergillosis is one of the most common invasive fungal infections and is often associated with high morbidity and mortality.

Most common sites of involvement are cutaneous, naso-orbital, pulmonary, and CNS; at times the infection could be disseminated. Invasive pulmonary aspergillosis occurs more commonly in immunocompromised individuals and presents as pneumonia. Major immunocompromised states for invasive pulmonary aspergillosis include HIV/AIDS, neutropenia, hematologic malignancies, chemotherapy, and prolonged use of immunosuppressive agents such as in bone marrow and solid organ transplant recipients. Hematogenous dissemination involving the CNS, heart, GIT, kidneys, liver, and spleen may occur in 25–33 % profoundly immunosuppressed patients.

Demonstration of fungal hyphae in tissues is diagnostic of invasive fungal infection. On light microscopic examination, *Aspergillus* reveals septate dichotomously branching (acute angles at 45°) hyphae with parallel walls 3–6 μm in diameter, there is minimal or no constriction at the septae. On HE stain, the hyphae appear basophilic to amphophilic, and PAS and GSM stains demonstrate the fungus well. Direct fluorescent antibodies can be applied for definitive identification. Culture identification of causative species is required for deciding appropriate antifungal therapy.

Aspergillus Abscess of the Palm in a Patient on Prolonged Steroid Therapy

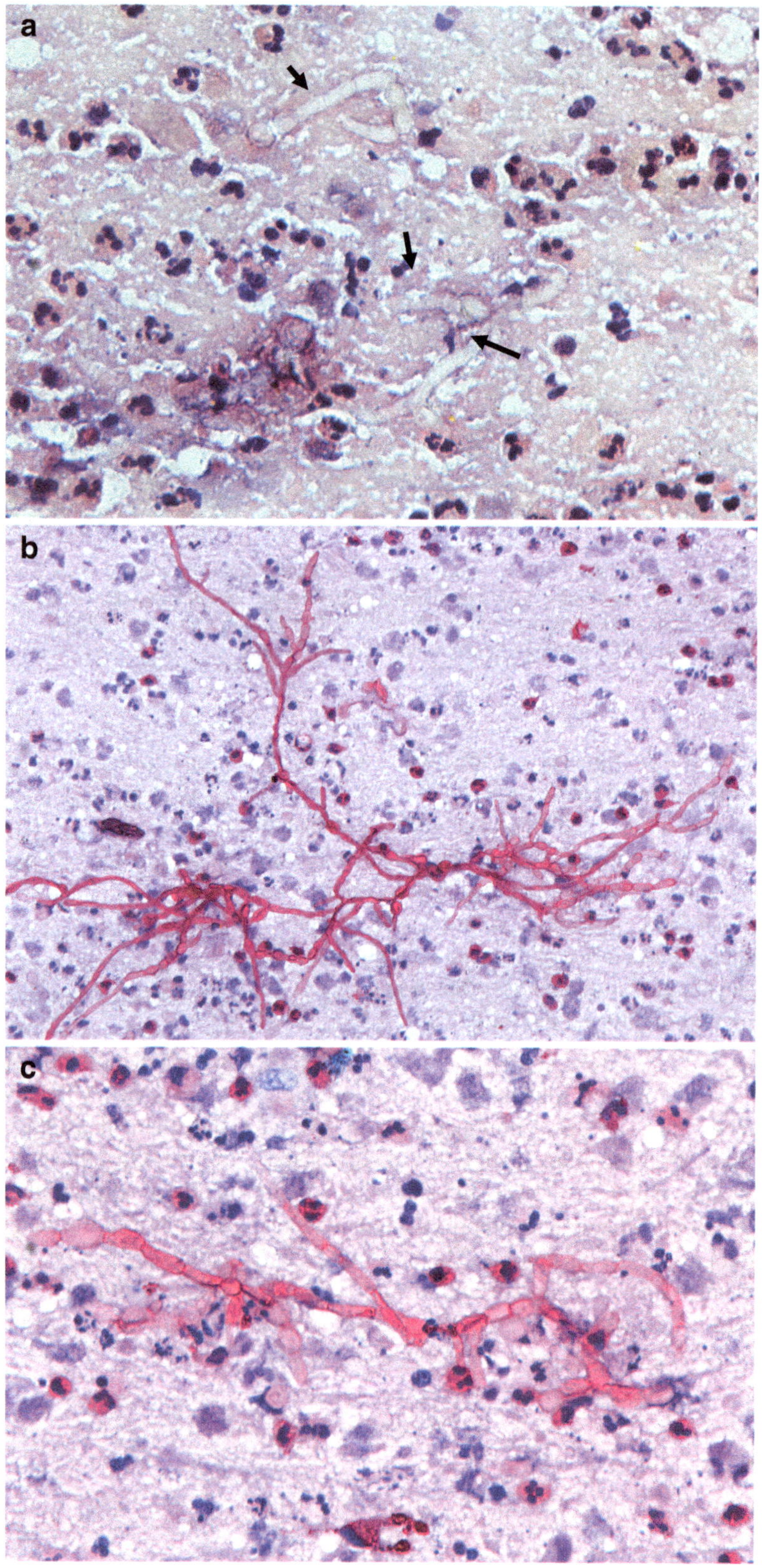

Fig. 4.24 (**a–c**) A 59-year-old male patient presented with hypertension for 7 years. About 3 months ago, he had undergone CABG for CAD. He was nondiabetic and nonsmoker. For about 8 years, he was on steroid therapy for IgA nephropathy. He presented with hematuria, mild proteinuria, and mild pedal edema for 2 weeks; he also had a swelling in the left palm for 10 days which was tender. FNAC from the swelling in the palm showed thin parallel-walled septate obtuse angle branching fungal hyphae along with club-shaped vesicles forming chains of conidia (**a** MGG ×400 negative staining-*arrow*), **b** PAS ×200, and **c** PAS ×400)

Aspergillus in Ulcer Foot in a Diabetic Renal Allograft Recipient

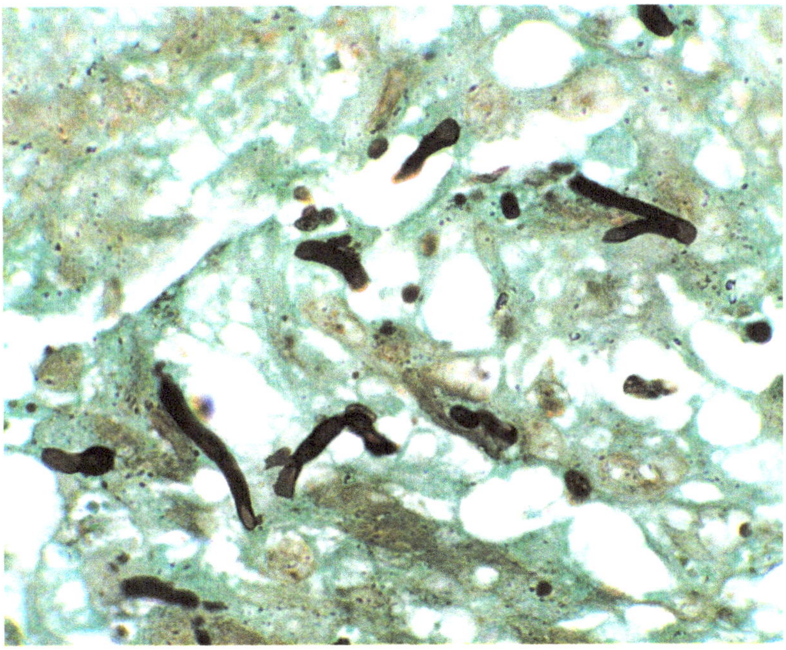

Fig. 4.25 A 61-year-old male diabetic patient receiving live-related renal allograft (primary disease diabetic nephropathy) presented with a nonhealing ulcer measuring 4 × 4 cm over the middle of the right sole. Biopsy from the ulcer showed fragmented but thin and parallel-walled acute angle branching hyphae of *Aspergillus* (CSM ×400) (From: Gupta RK. In *Pathology of opportunistic infections in tropic*. Jaypee; 2007)

Aspergillus in Ankle Swelling in a Renal Allograft Recipient

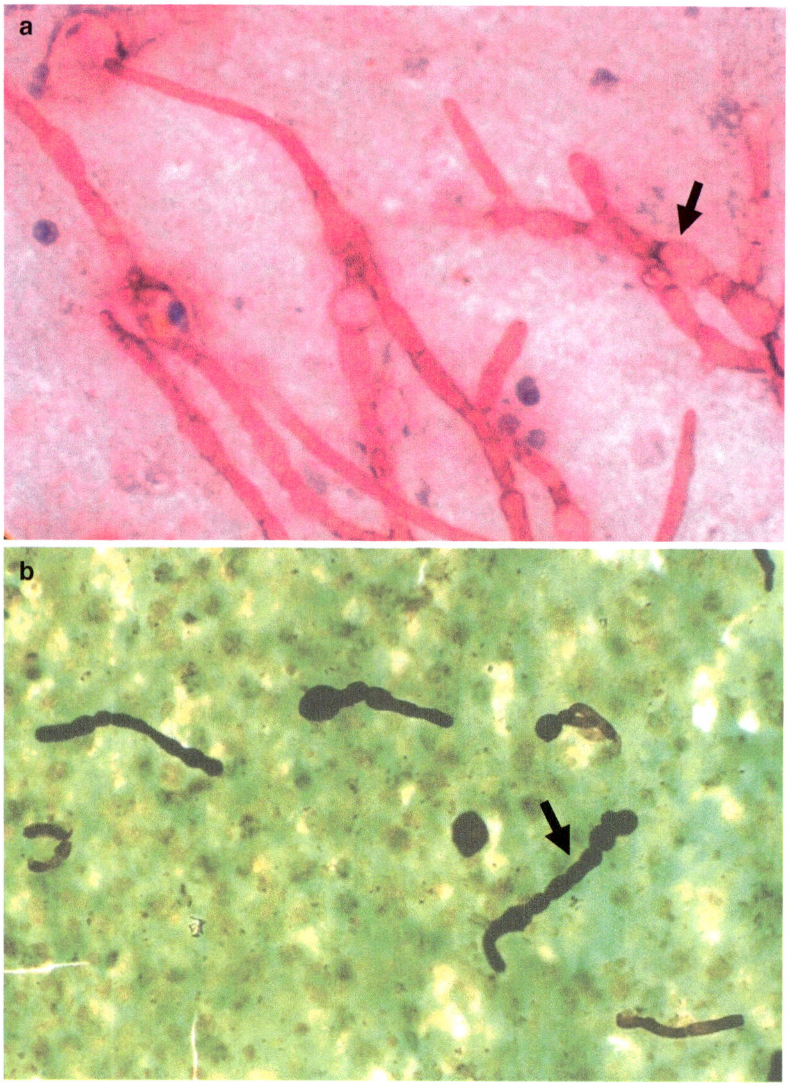

Fig. 4.26 (**a**, **b**) A 40-year-old male patient receiving live-related renal allograft developed swelling of the right ankle 1 year posttransplant. Fine-needle aspiration cytology from the swelling showed uniform septate acute angle branching fungal hyphae with club-shaped vesicles forming chains of conidia (*arrow*) suggestive of *Aspergillus* (**a** PAS ×400, **b** CSM ×400) (From: Gupta RK. In *Pathology of opportunistic infections in tropic*. Jaypee; 2007)

Nasal Aspergillosis in a Patient of AML

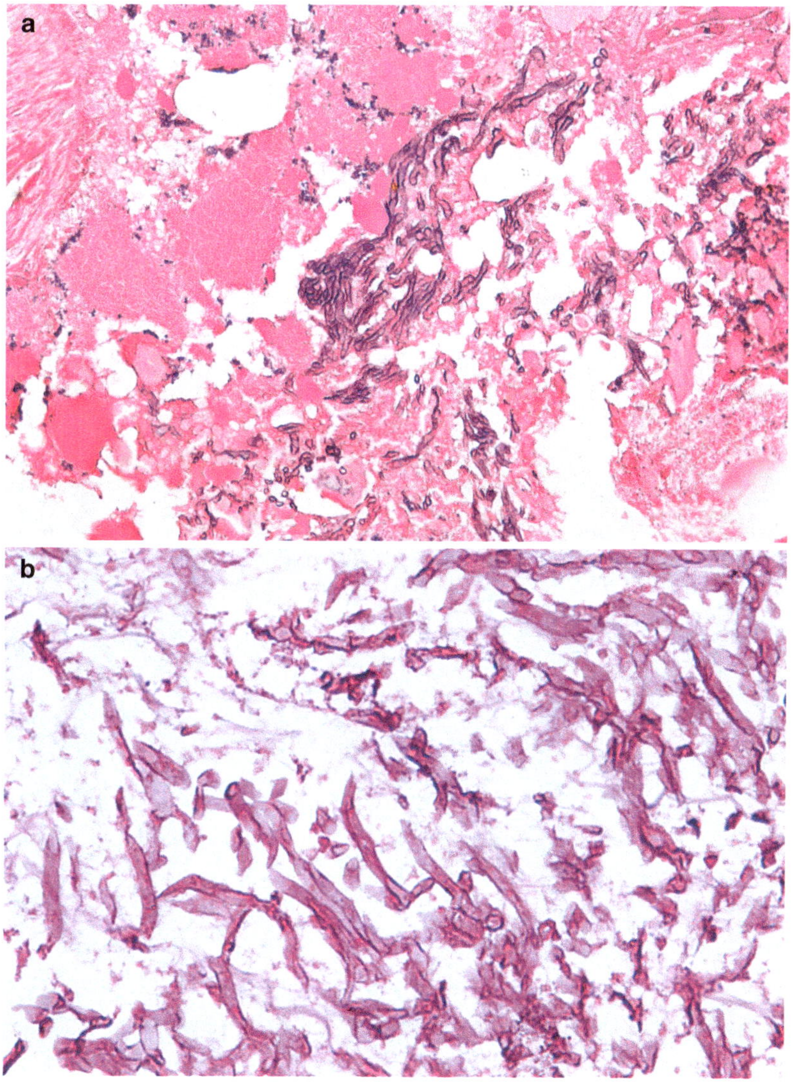

Fig. 4.27 (**a**, **b**) A 23-year-old female patient, a known case of AML in remission after recently being treated with high-dose cytarabine, developed bilateral nasal obstruction, more so on the left side. CT showed bilateral maxillary sinusitis. She sneezed out some necrotic material. The histological examination showed plenty of thin parallel-walled septate obtuse angle branching hyphae of *Aspergillus* (**a** HE ×200, **b** PAS ×400)

Aspergillus in Sputum in a Patient of ALL

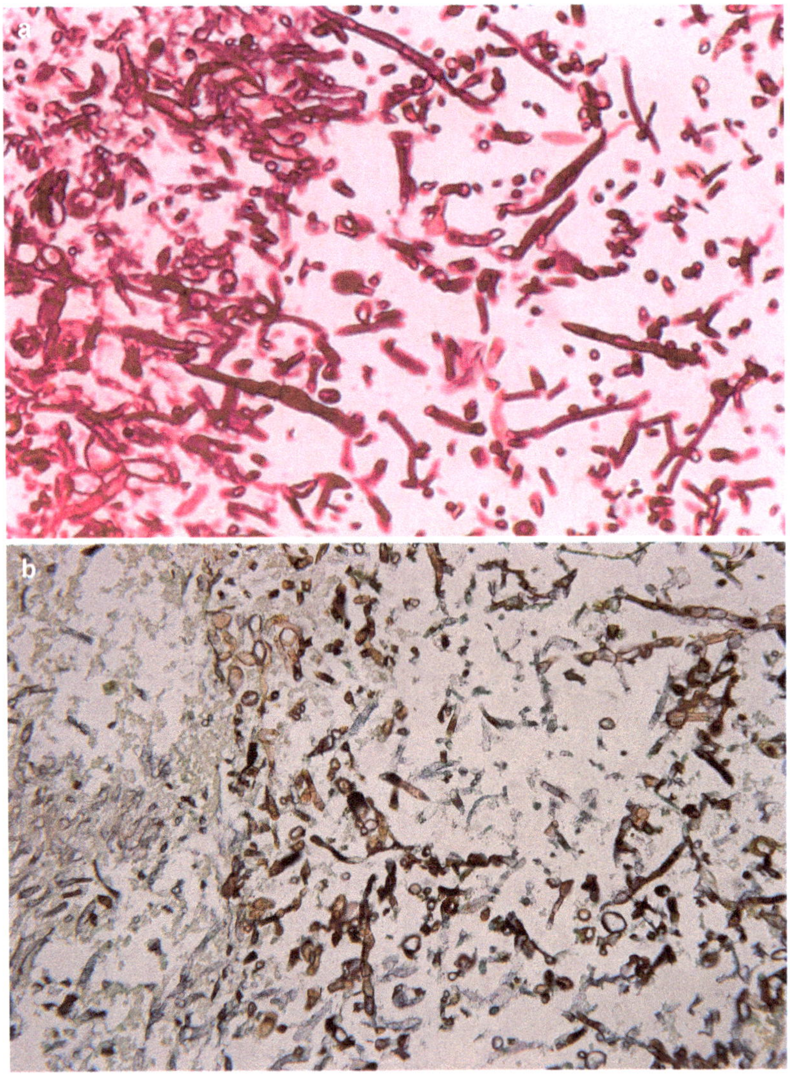

Fig. 4.28 (**a**, **b**) A 25-year-old male patient on chemotherapy for ALL presented with dyspnea and bilateral basal crepts. Coughed out material on histopathological evaluation revealed acute angle branching septate hyphae of *Aspergillus*. (**a** PAS ×400, **b** CSM ×400) (From: Gupta RK. In *Pathology of opportunistic infections in tropic*. Jaypee; 2007)

Aspergillosis Lung in a Renal Allograft Recipient

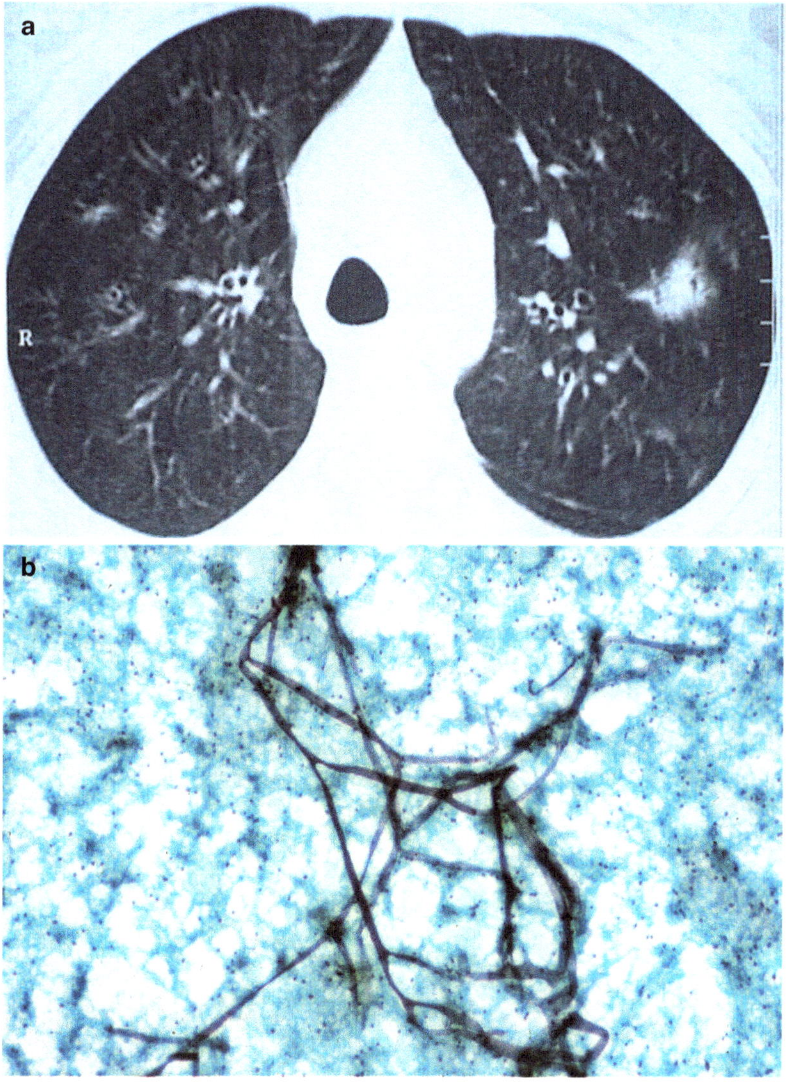

Fig. 4.29 (**a**, **b**) A 36-year-old male patient received live-related renal allograft 10 years back and was maintained on wysolone and azaron. He presented with fever, cough, and breathlessness for 15 days. Chest CT revealed multiple bilateral consolidations (**a**). He underwent bronchoscopy; bronchoalveolar lavage (BAL) showed long acute angle branching filamentous hyphae suggestive of *Aspergillus* (**b** GSM ×200) (Contributor – Dr. S Radha, Aware Global Hospital, Hyderabad, India)

Bronchial Aspergillosis in a Diabetic Patient

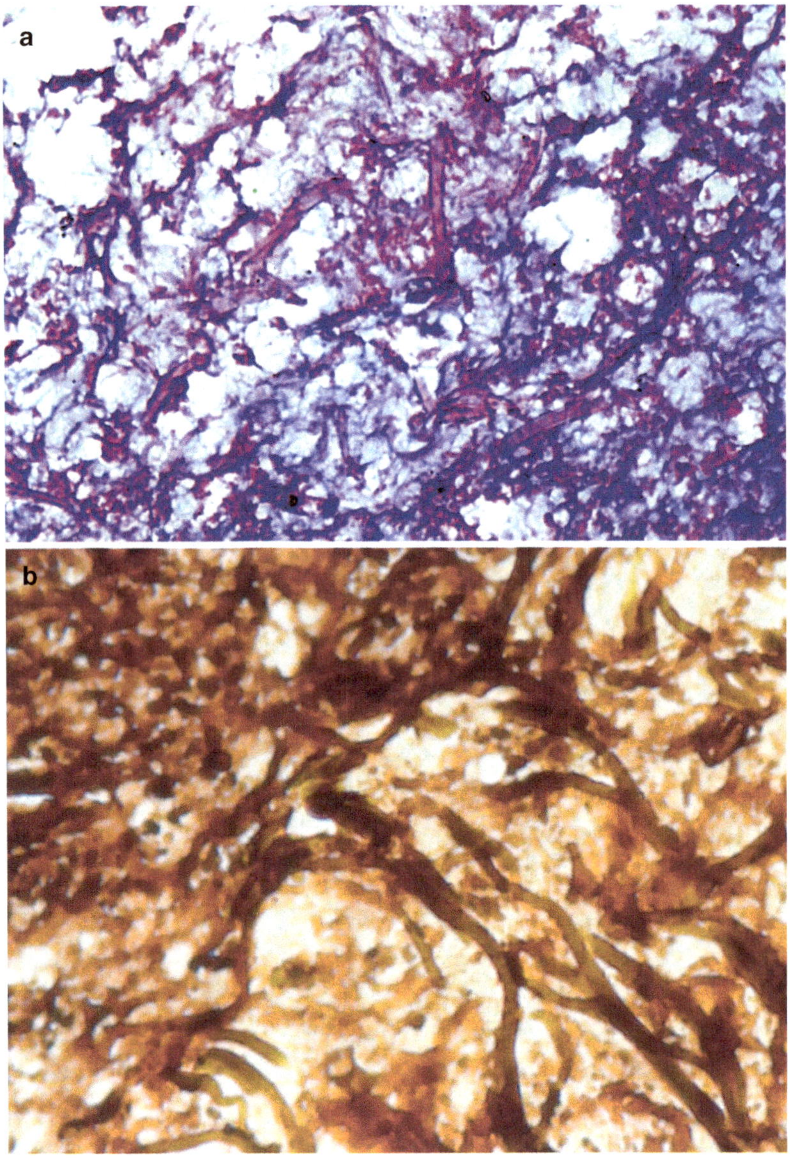

Fig. 4.30 (**a**, **b**) A 48-year-old female diabetic patient, who had been receiving corticosteroids for chronic obstructive lung disease, presented with fever and breathlessness. Chest X-ray revealed bilateral lobar pneumonia. She was ventilated and received broad-spectrum antibiotics to which she partially responded. Bronchoscopy revealed necrotic debris obstructing the bronchioles. The bronchoscopic aspiration revealed plenty of parallel thin-walled, septate, acute angle branching fungal hyphae suggestive of *Aspergillus* (**a** PAS ×400, and **b** CSM ×400)

Pleural Aspergillosis in an Elderly Chronically Ill Patient of Thoracic Empyema

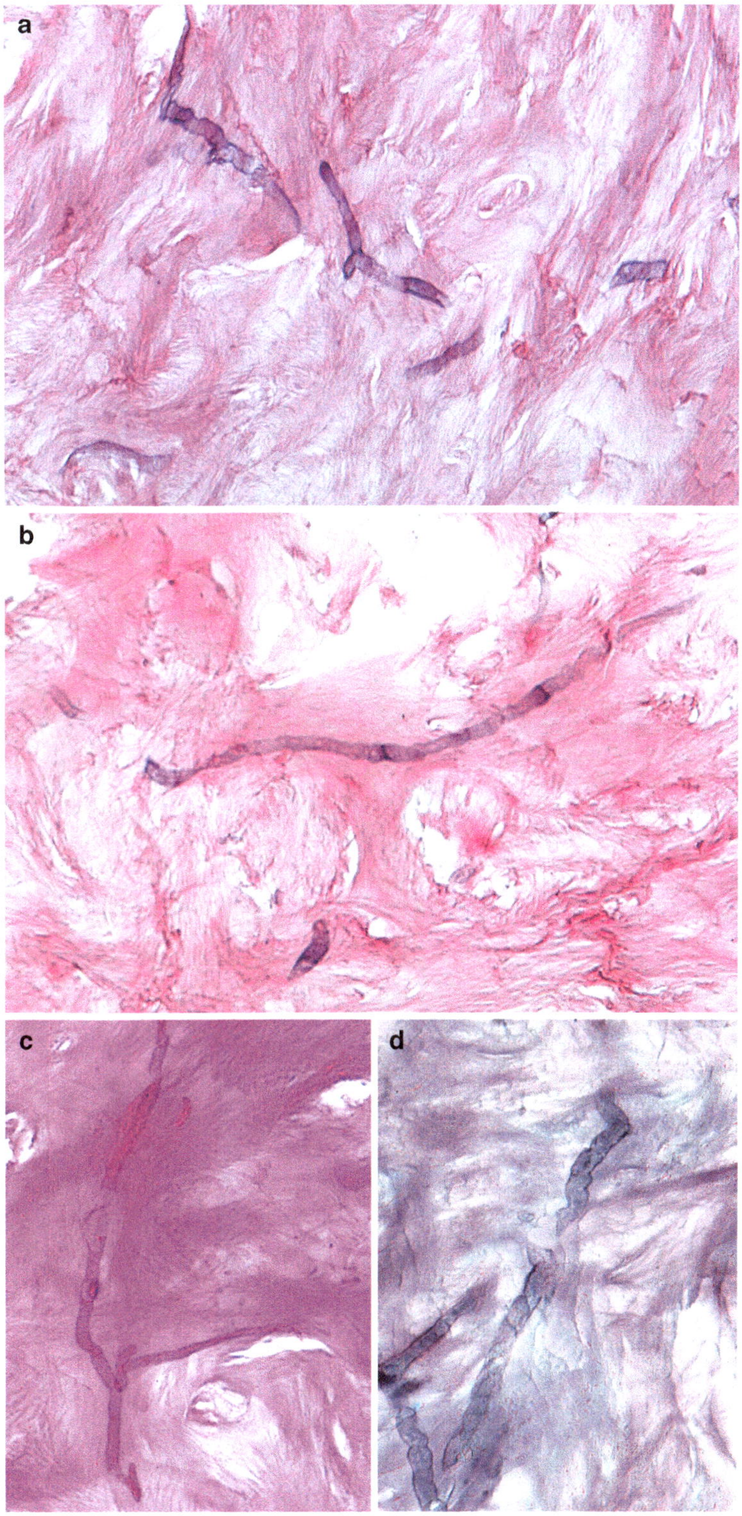

Fig. 4.31 (**a–d**) A 70-year-old male patient presented with pyrexia and difficulty in breathing and left-sided chest pain for 6 weeks. Clinical examination revealed dullness and reduced air entry in the left middle and lower zone with the presence of basal crepts. He had past history (about 15 years back) of treated pulmonary tuberculosis. Cardiac workup revealed minimal pericardial effusion and right bundle branch block (RBBB), and the ejection fraction was 55 %. Chest X-ray showed encysted empyema with thickened pleura on the left side of the chest. Laboratory workup revealed mild anemia (Hb 10.1 g/dl), and total WBC count was 11,300/cu mm with 68 % neutrophils. He had hypoalbuminemia with serum albumin being 1.13 g/dl. He was nondiabetic. Liver function and kidney function tests were WNL. Intercostal drain was placed which yielded thick purulent material. In view of continuous purulent discharge, the ICD had to be placed for more than 6 months, when thoracotomy with decortication was performed. Thoracotomy revealed encysted thoracic empyema; the pleura was found to be markedly thickened and calcified. Histological examination of the pleura revealed areas of necrosis along with few septate fungal hyphae having thin parallel walls, with acute angle branching, suggestive of *Aspergillus* (**a**, **b** HE ×400, **c** PAS ×400 and **d** CSM ×400)

Meningeal Aspergilloma in a Patient with Recurrent Infections

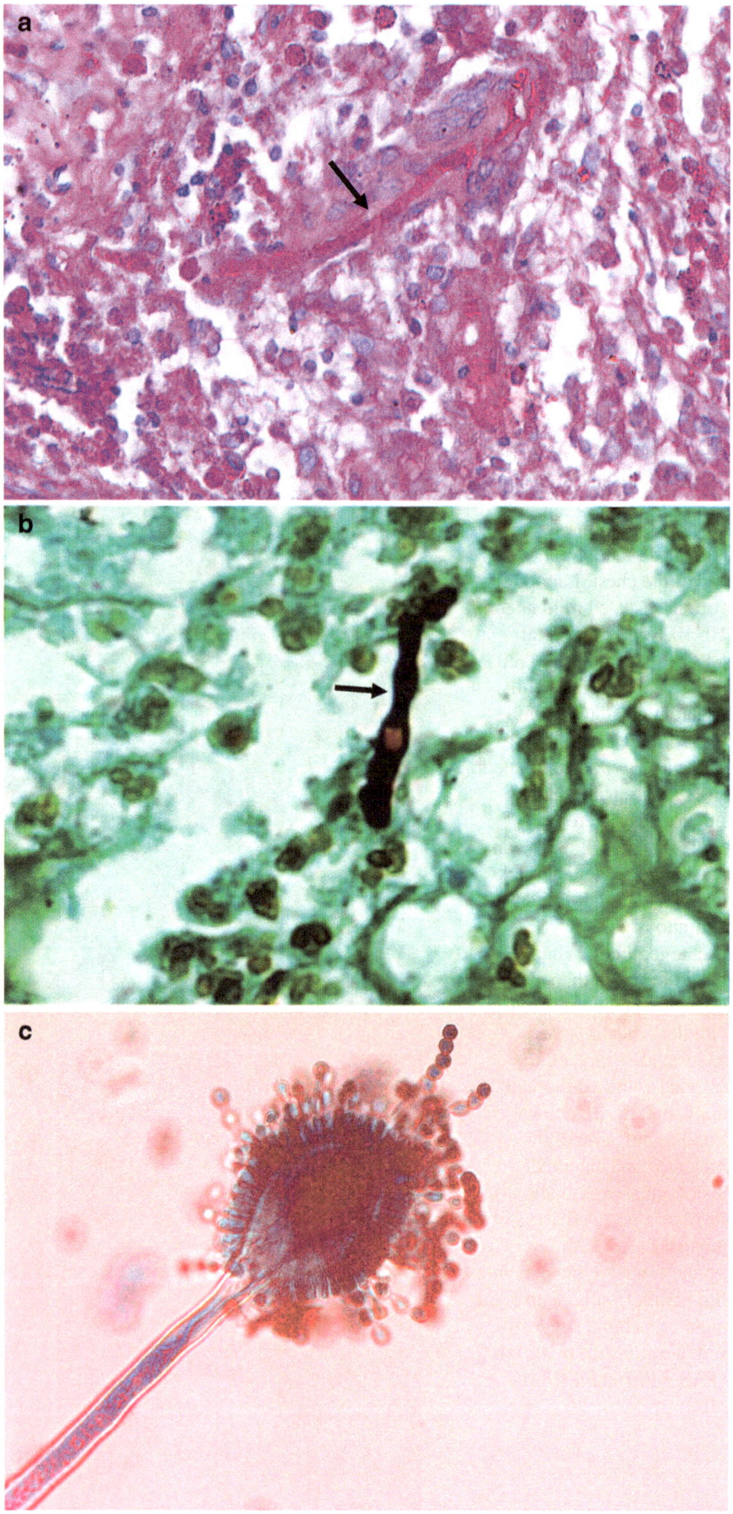

Fig. 4.32 (**a–c**) A 21-year-old male patient presented with mild to moderate holocranial headache for 2 months followed by progressive loss of vision in both eyes for 1 month. The patient had history of recurrent sinusitis. MRI revealed moderate-sized homogeneously enhancing well-defined elongated and lobulated anterior skull base, extra-axial soft tissue space-occupying lesion with suprasellar and intrasellar extension. Extensive ethmoid and sphenoid sinusitis was evident. Total WBC count was 11,500/cu mm with 23 % eosinophils. At surgery, a yellowish grey mass was seen originating from the dura. Histopathological examination showed multiple giant cell granulomas along with plenty of fungal profiles having thin parallel-walled septate hyphae having chains of small club-shaped conidia of *Aspergillus*. Slide culture for fungus showed hyaline, branched, septate hyphae with fruiting heads borne on long sporangiophores. Spores are borne on biseriate sterigma covering full area of globose columella, characteristic of *Aspergillus* sp. (**a** PAS ×400, **b** CSM ×400 and **c** Lactophenol Cotton *Blue* ×400) (Contributor to mycological workup: Dr. Vipul Kumar Srivastava, Consultant Microbiologist, Sahara Hospital, Lucknow, India)

Meningeal Aspergillosis in a Postoperative Patient

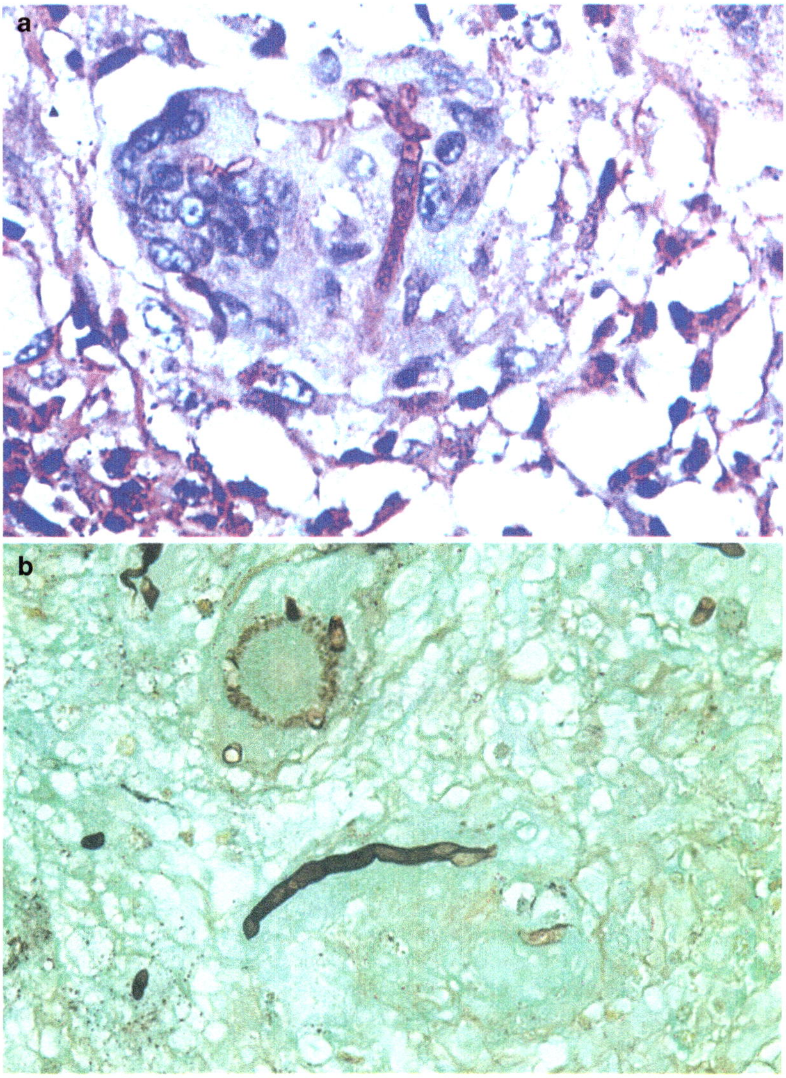

Fig. 4.33 (**a–b**) A 45-year-old female patient presented to a peripheral hospital with chief complaints of headache and seizures of 3 weeks duration. Cranial CT revealed a left frontotemporal dural-based SOL. Craniotomy was performed, and a mengingeal tumor was excised which on histopathological examination was found to be meningothelial meningioma. Postoperative recovery was uneventful. However, 3 months later, she again presented with headache for 2 weeks along with weakness of the right upper and lower limb for 2 days. The lab parameters were within normal limits. The cranial CT revealed hyperdense extra-axial enhancing mass in the left basifrontal region measuring 37 × 16 × 38 mm. Clinical diagnosis of recurrent meningioma was made, craniotomy was performed, and the mass was excised. The histopathological examination of the mass revealed granulomatous inflammatory lesion with the presence of both foreign body and Langhans giant cells along with the presence of thin parallel-walled septate hyphae having chains of small club-shaped conidia both within and outside the giant cells, suggestive of meningeal aspergilloma (**a** PAS ×400, **b** CSM ×400)

Aspergillus in Brain Abscess in a Diabetic Renal Allograft Recipient

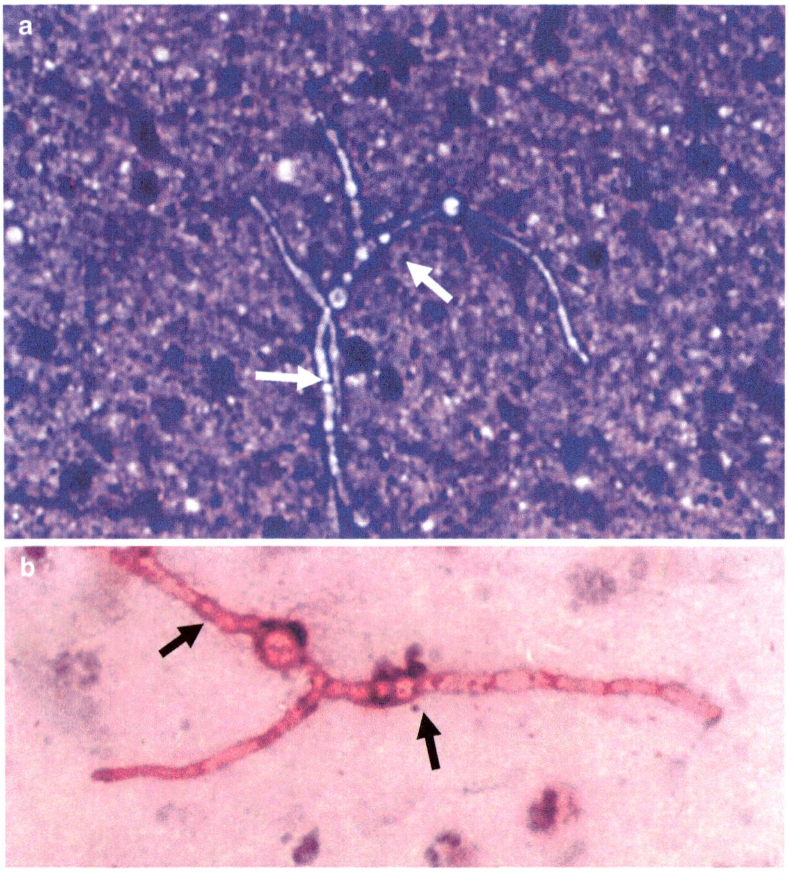

Fig. 4.34 (**a**, **b**) A 52-year-old diabetic renal allograft recipient 3 years posttransplant presented with delirium and epileptic attacks for 10 days. Skull CT showed a 3 × 3 cm space-occupying mass in the left frontal lobe. At craniotomy, tissue from the suspected area was subjected for rapid intraoperative cytological evaluation. Imprint smears showed glial tissue infiltrated with septate obtuse angle branching thin parallel-walled hyphae along with club-shaped vesicles forming chains of conidia (*arrows*) of *Aspergillus* (**a** MGG ×400, **b** PAS ×400)

Aspergillosis of the Brain (Post Chicken Pox)

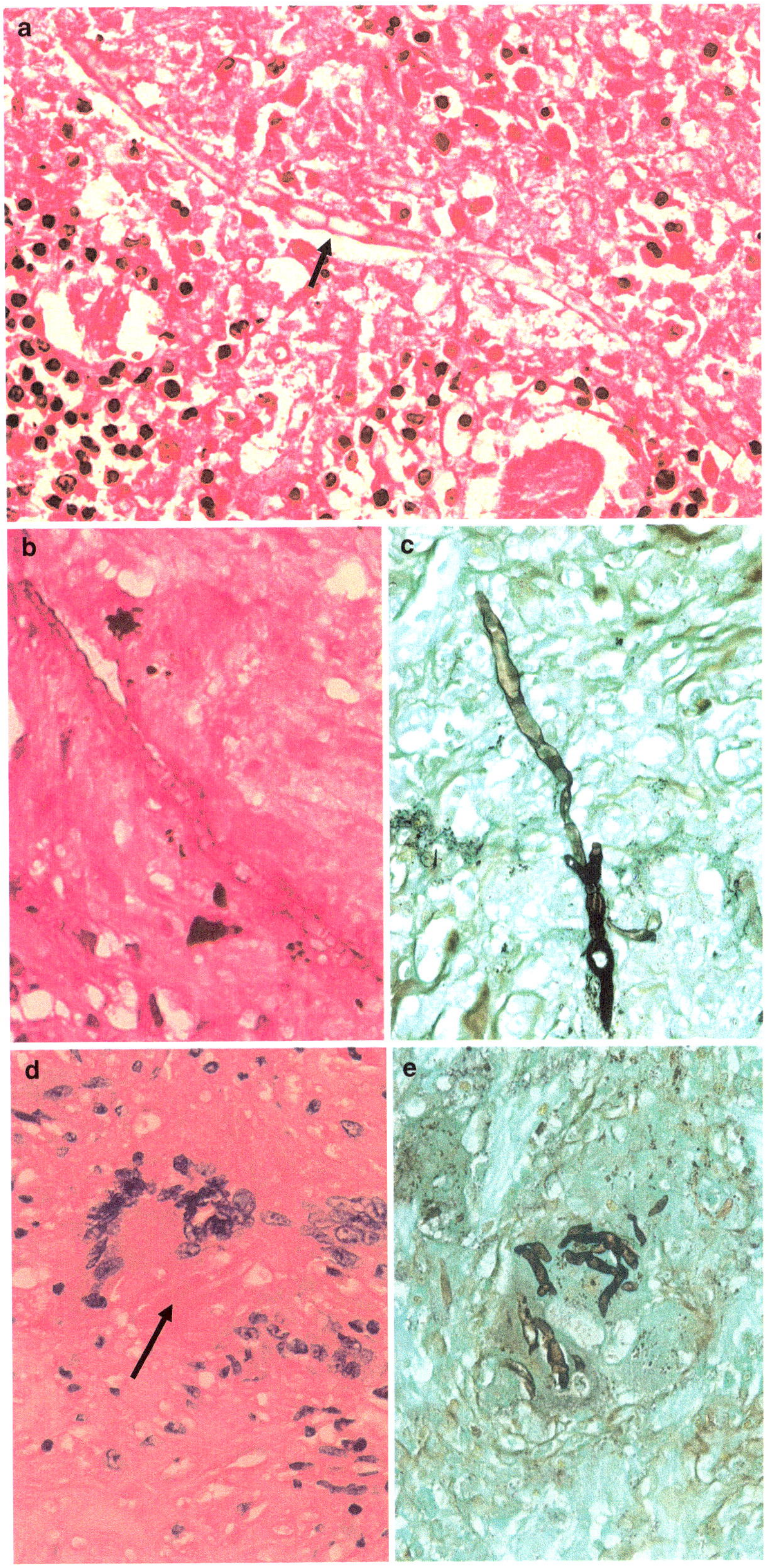

Fig. 4.35 (**a**–**e**) A 32-year-old female patient with past history of chicken pox a month ago presented with recurrent seizures and altered sensorium for 15 days and unconsciousness for 1 day. Cranial CT revealed frontotemporal SOL. Right frontotemporal decompressive craniotomy with the excision of SOL was performed. The histopathological examination showed widespread necrosis of brain parenchyma with polymorphonuclear inflammatory infiltrate along with a few foreign body giant cells and slender septate fungal hyphae with thin parallel walls and acute angle branching; oval or spherical chlamydospores were also seen (**a** HE ×400, **b** PAS ×400, **c** CSM ×400). The fungal elements were also identified within the giant cells (**d** HE ×400 negative stain – *arrow*) and (**e** CSM ×400)

Zygomycetes (Causative Agent of Zygomycosis, Phycomycosis, and Mucormycosis): Zygomycetes are present as natural flora of soil and decaying organic matter. Infection is acquired through inhalation of sporangiospores or through ingestion of contaminated food. Commonly encountered manifestations are rhinocerebral, pulmonary, gastrointestinal, cutaneous, and disseminated. The characteristic feature of this class of fungi is their property of angioinvasion resulting in hematogenous spread. Disseminated infection may involve any organ.

Biopsy, nasal scrapings, scrapings of cutaneous lesions, fine-needle aspirates of paranasal mass, bronchoalveolar lavage, gastric aspirates, feces, or sputum as the case be may show the fungal elements. The fungal hyphae are broad (6–25 μm), irregular in width, thick walled, and aseptate, branching at right angles. Clamydospores (15–30 μm) are thick-walled spherical to oval structures appearing as empty rings in tissue sections. Fungal hyphae stain light basophilic to amphophilic on HE. PAS and GSM stains are useful in demonstration of fungal elements. The presence of characteristic fungal elements in tissue sections is diagnostic. Direct immunofluorescence can be applied to paraffin sections for species identification. Culture identification is required for the demonstration of specific fungal pathogens.

The fungus characteristically invades the blood vessels causing thrombosis, infarction, and hemorrhage. Invasive zygomycosis spreads rapidly causing severe morbidity and mortality. Early and prompt diagnosis and institution of appropriate antifungal therapy is essential for better outcome in these patients.

Table 4.3 Differentiating morphological features of common filamentous fungi

Features	*Aspergillus*	Zygomycetes
Width	Narrow (3–6 μm)	Broad (6–25 μm)
Appearance	Uniform/parallel walls	Nonuniform/nonparallel
Branching	Regular, dichotomous, acute angles	Irregular, right angles
Septation	Present	Absent
Chlamydoconidia	Absent[a]	Present
CMS/PAS staining	Strong positive	Weak positive

From: Gupta RK. In *Pathology of opportunistic infections in tropic*. Jaypee; 2007
[a]Conidial heads may form in cavitory lesions.

Zygomycosis of the Lung in a Renal Allograft Recipient

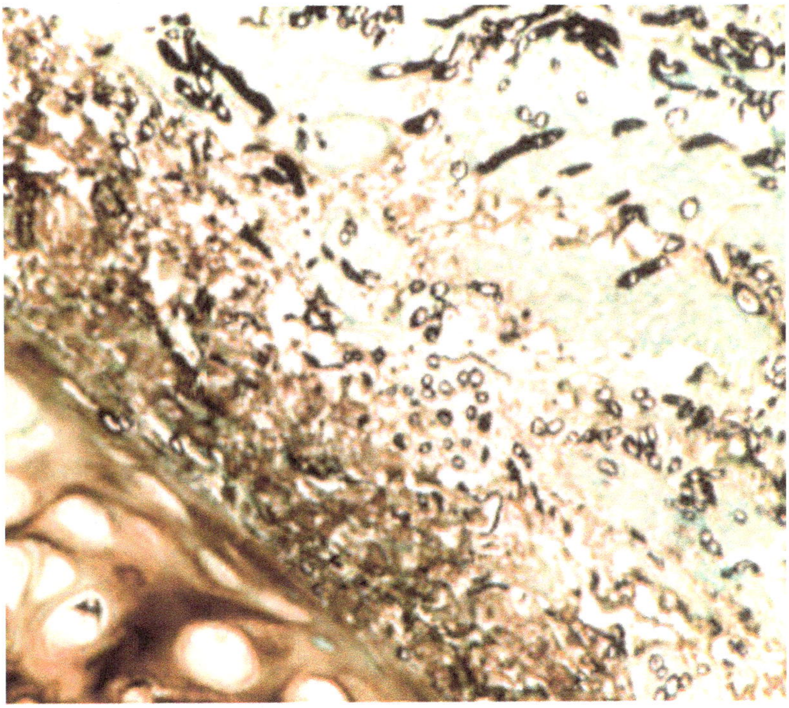

Fig. 4.36 A 56-year-old male patient receiving live-related renal allograft, 2 years posttransplant presented with high-grade fever, recent onset dyspnea, and watery stools. The patient was cyanotic and had bilateral diffuse rhonchi. Hematological profile revealed agranulocytosis. He died soon after hospitalization. Postmortem lung biopsy showed necrotic tissue infiltrated with broad aseptate irregularly branching fungal hyphae (in longitudinal cuts; in transverse cuts, the fungal hyphae appear as thick-walled rings) suggestive of zygomycosis (CSM ×400) (From: Gupta RK. In *Pathology of opportunistic infections in tropic*. Jaypee; 2007)

Disseminated Zygomycosis Involving Maxillary Sinus and Colon in a Renal Allograft Recipient

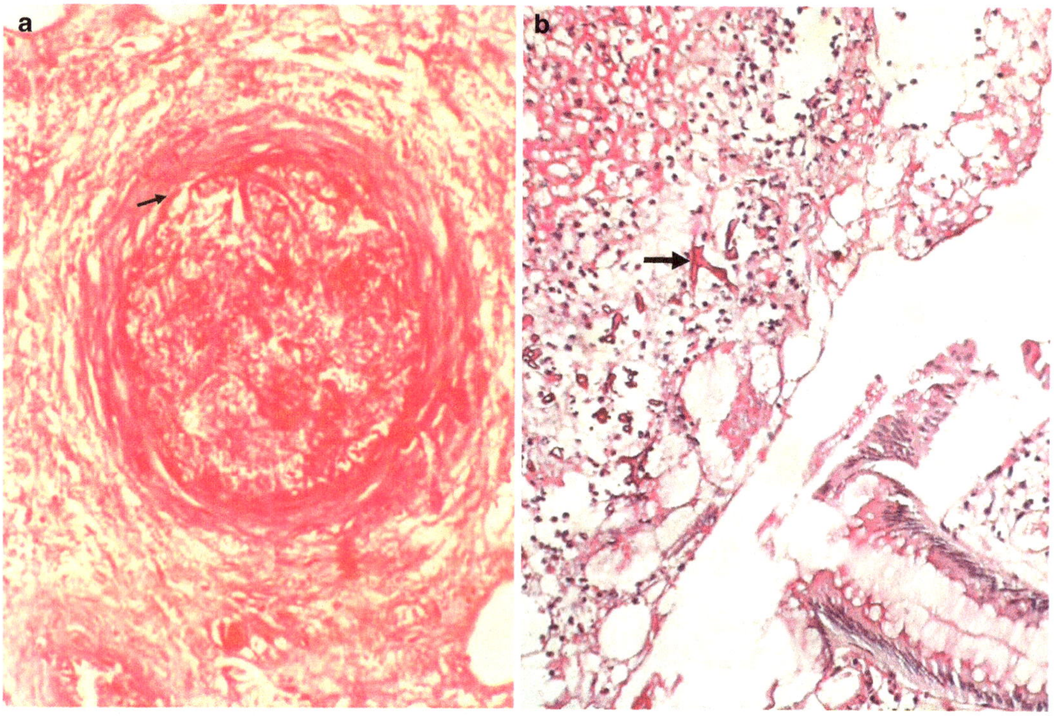

Fig. 4.37 (**a**, **b**) A 60-year-old male patient receiving live-related renal allograft, 6 months posttransplant, presented with left-sided headache, sinusitis, and weakness; subsequently he developed 6th and 7th nerve palsy and colonic perforation. Biopsy from maxillary sinus showed broad aseptate fungal hyphae with angioinvasion (*arrow*) (**a** HE ×400). Biopsy from colonic perforation also showed similar fungal elements (*arrow*) (**b** PAS ×400) suggestive of disseminated zygomycosis (From: Gupta RK. In *Pathology of opportunistic infections in tropic*. Jaypee; 2007)

Zygomycosis Renal Allograft

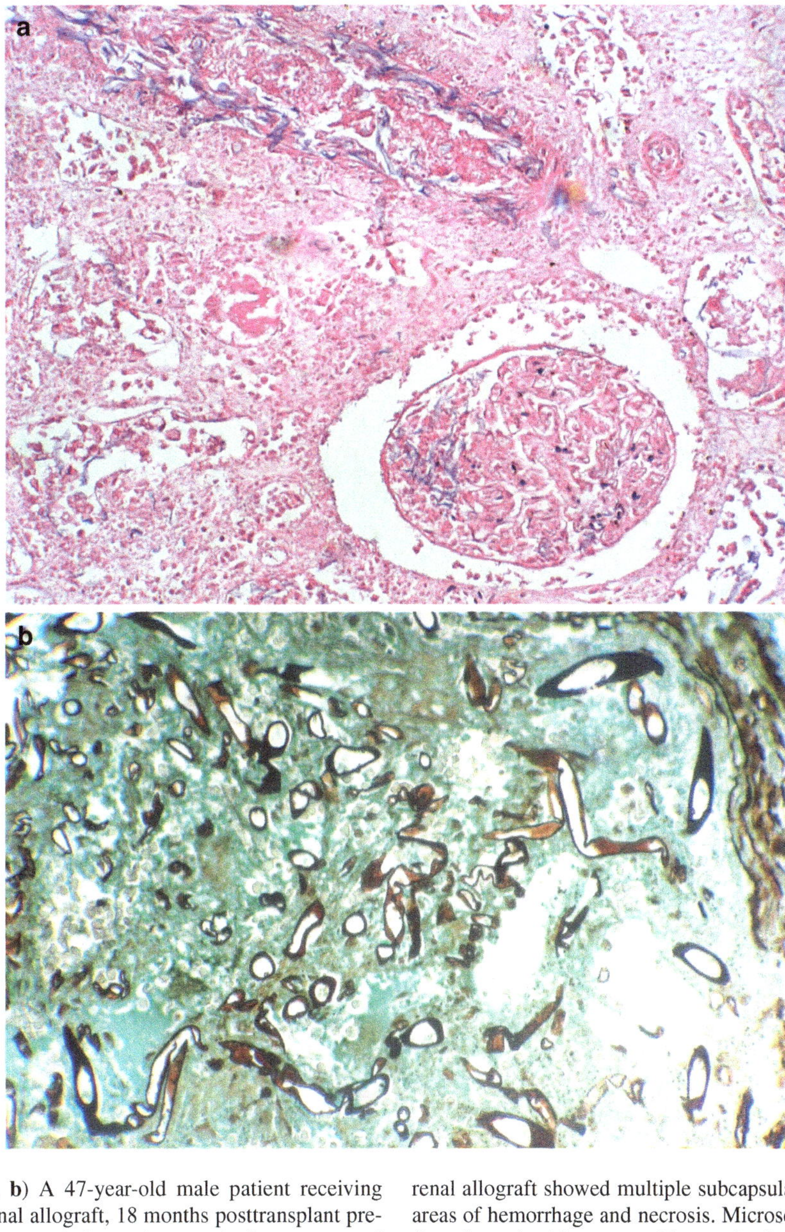

Fig. 4.38 (**a**, **b**) A 47-year-old male patient receiving live-related renal allograft, 18 months posttransplant presented with high-grade fever, decreased urine output, and rising serum creatinine. Ultrasonographic examination revealed markedly swollen and enlarged graft with complete loss of corticomedullary details. Soon the patient developed advanced renal failure, and graft nephrectomy had to be performed. Gross examination of explanted renal allograft showed multiple subcapsular infarcts with areas of hemorrhage and necrosis. Microscopic examination showed wide areas of hemorrhagic necrosis infiltrated with irregular, broad, and aseptate fungal hyphae having wide-angle branching and prominent angioinvasion. The diagnosis of zygomycosis was offered (**a** HE ×400 and **b** CSM ×400) (From: Gupta RK. In *Pathology of opportunistic infections in tropic*. Jaypee; 2007)

Zygomycosis in Gluteal Abscess in a Patient of ALL

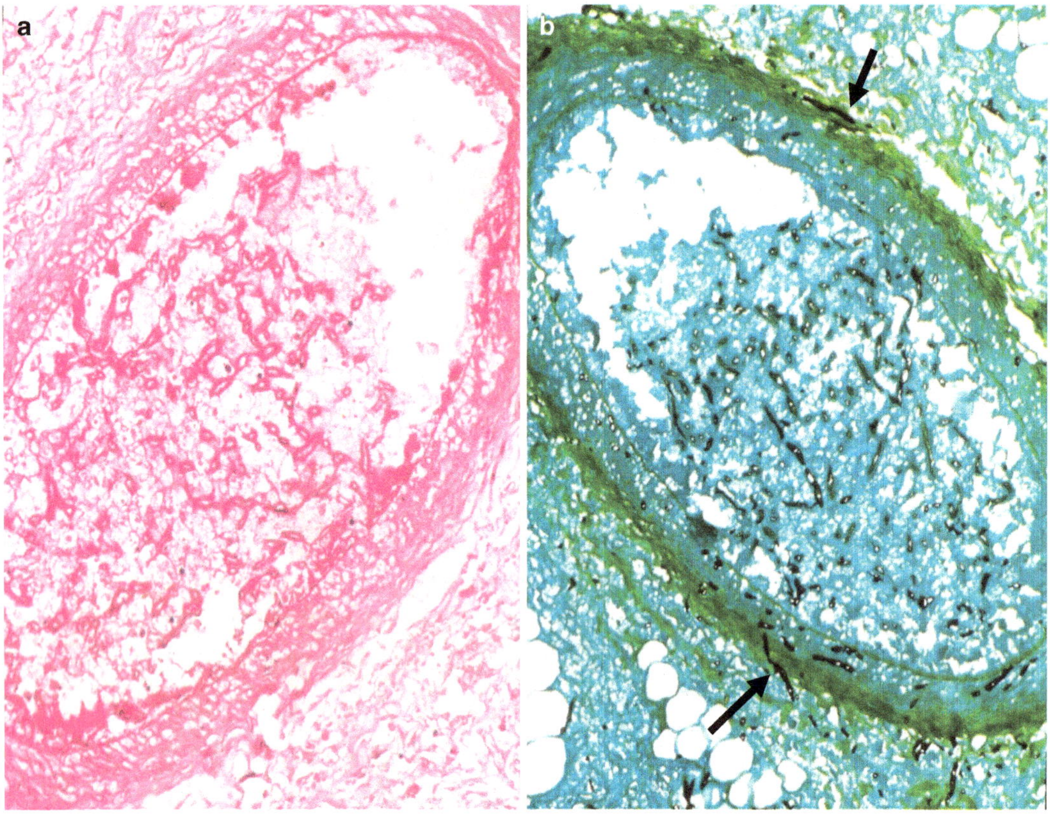

Fig. 4.39 (**a**, **b**) A 14-year-old male patient known to have been suffering from ALL presented with gluteal abscess. Histopathological examination of the tissue obtained from abscess wall revealed extensive necrosis and hemorrhage along with angioinvasion (*arrow*) with broad aseptate fungal hyphae suggestive of zygomycosis. (**a** PAS ×200 and **b** CSM ×200) (From: Gupta RK. In *Pathology of opportunistic infections in tropic*. Jaypee; 2007)

Orbital Zygomycosis in a Diabetic Patient

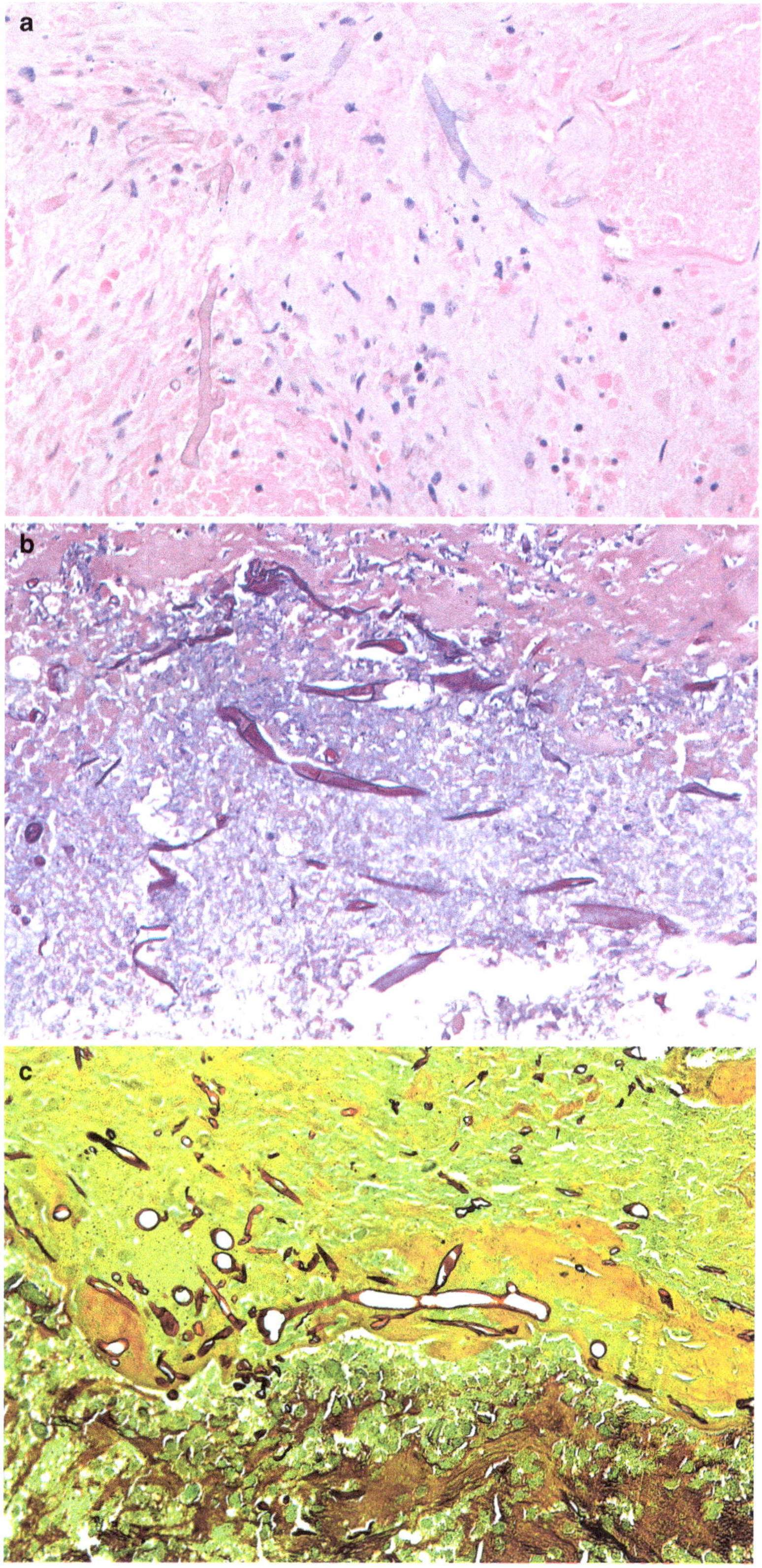

Fig. 4.40 (**a**–**e**) A 62-year-old female diabetic patient who was on insulin therapy presented with a left ethmoidal mass with orbital extension and involvement of orbital apex. She was found to have total ophthalmoplegia with optic nerve compression. Orbital exenteration with external ethmoidectomy was performed. Histological examination of the orbital contents predominantly showed necrosis with granulomatous inflammation and numerous foreign body giant cells along with irregular, broad thick-walled partially septate fungal hyphae invading the blood vessels suggestive of invasive zygomycosis (**a** HE ×400, **b** PAS ×400, **c** CSM ×400); optic nerve also showed invasion with similar fungal hyphae **d** HE ×400 and **e** CSM ×400)

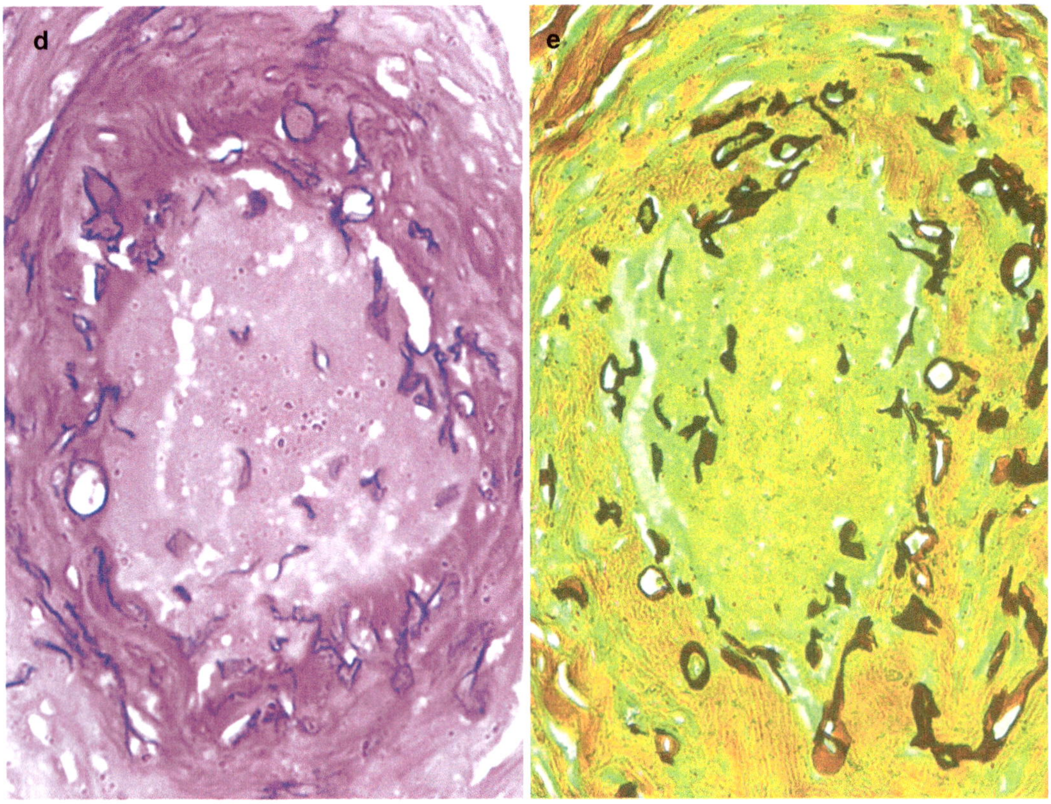

Fig. 4.40 (continued)

Zygomycosis of the Brain After VPLP Shunting

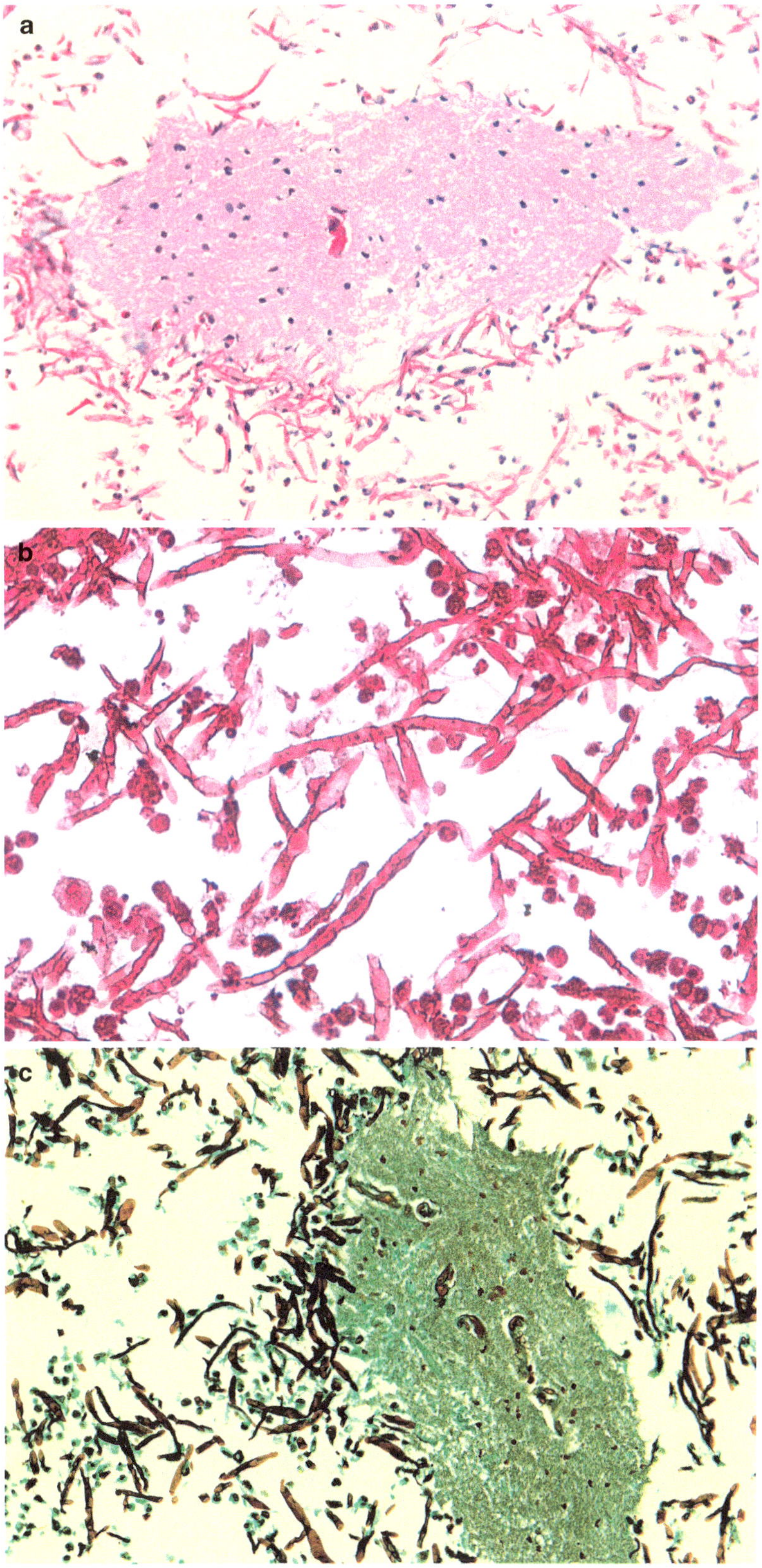

Fig. 4.41 (**a**–**c**) A 22-year-old male patient presented with hydrocephalus consequent to tubercular meningitis. He was operated and a VPLP shunt was placed. However, the shunt failed, and the patient continued to have persistent headache and vomiting; he was, therefore, reexplored. The lateral ventricle was found to be occluded with granulation tissue, which was removed. The histopathological examination showed glial tissue infiltrated with polymorphonucelar inflammatory cells along with plenty of irregular and broad, right angle branching partially septate hyphae having club-shaped chlamydospores suggestive of cerebral zygomycosis (**a** PAS ×200, **b** PAS ×400 and **c** CSM ×200)

Mucormycosis in Nasal Polyp in a Diabetic Patient

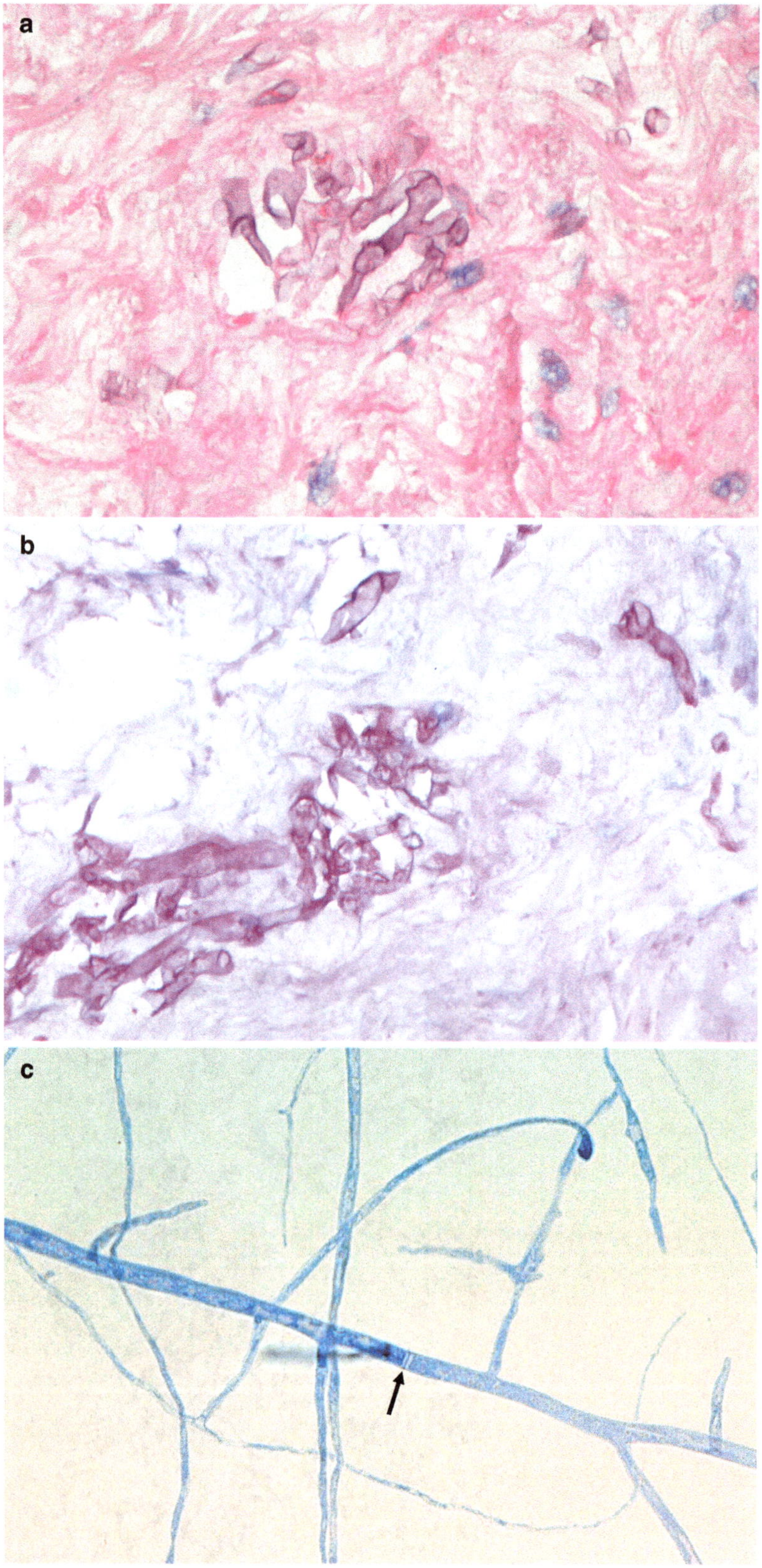

Fig. 4.42 (**a–d**) A 52-year-old diabetic female patient who had undergone coronary angioplasty using drug-eluting stent, 5 days later developed bilateral basal crepts, pericardial effusion with cardiac tamponade, and bilateral pleural effusion and septicemia necessitating ventilatory support. Laboratory workup revealed total WBC count of 34,100/cu mm having over 90 % neutrophils with a shift to the left. LFT revealed very high SGOT and SGPT levels (6989 IU/L and 15562 IU/L, respectively). Subsequently she also developed bilateral nasal polypoidal masses which were necrotic and friable. The histological examination of the biopsy obtained from the nasal mass showed necrotic tissue containing plenty of sparsely septate, broad, thick-walled irregular hyaline fungal hyphae suggestive of mucormycosis. Slide culture for fungus showed hyaline, branched, ribbon-shaped, and partially septate (*arrow*) hyphae along with mature and immature pear-shaped sporangia having hyaline sporangiospores with characteristic conical columella of *Absidia* sp. (**a** HE ×400, **b** PAS ×400 **c**, **d** Lactophenol cotton *blue* ×400) (Contributor to mycological workup – Dr. Vipul Kumar Srivastava, Consultant Microbiologist, Sahara Hospital, Lucknow, India)

Fig. 4.42 (continued)

d

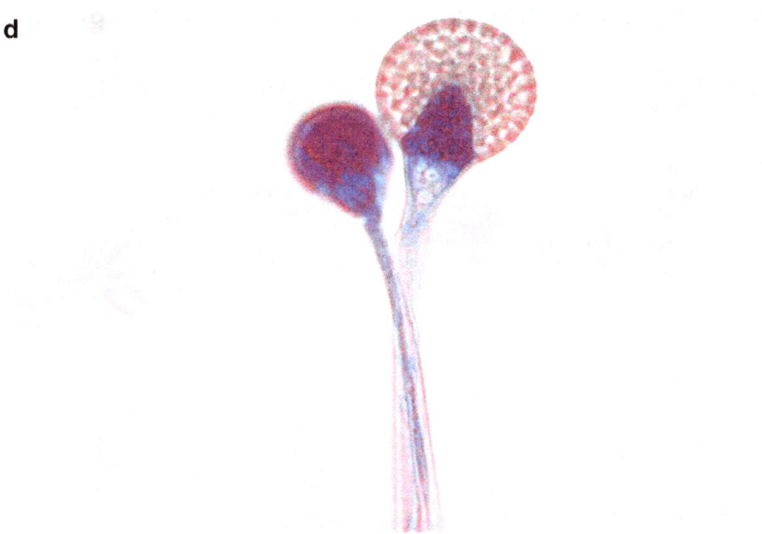

Mucormycosis of the Lung in a Renal Allograft Recipient

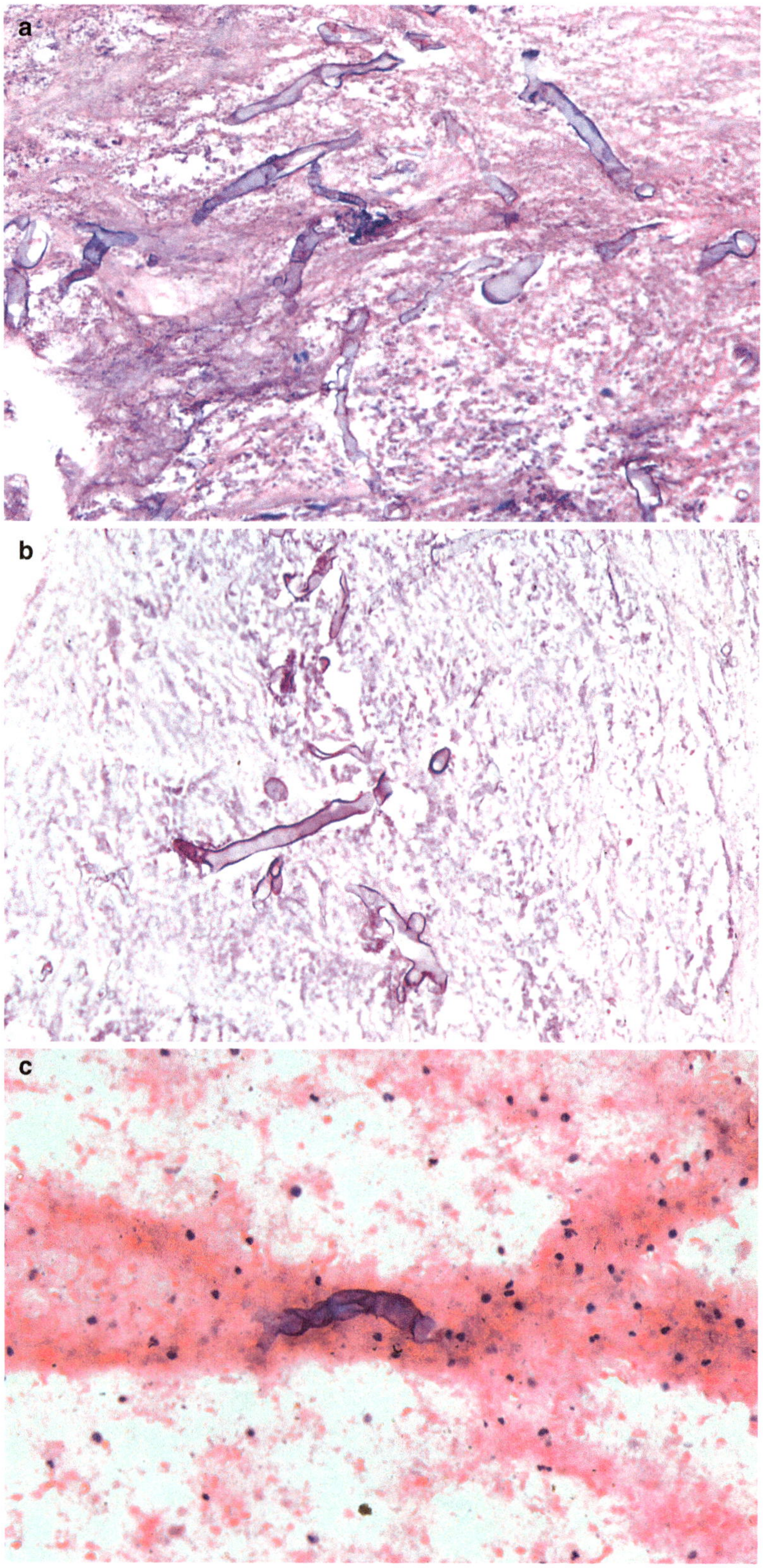

Fig. 4.43 (**a**–**c**) A 47-year-old male patient known to have been suffering with long-standing uncontrolled diabetes mellitus with end-stage diabetic kidney disease. He tested positive for HBsAg and anti-HCV. He received live-related renal allograft and was maintained on triple drug immunosuppression. Subsequently 20 months posttransplant, he presented with fever and cough for 15 days. Clinical evaluation revealed right upper lobe consolidation, and CT-guided FNAC showed mucormycosis; fungal culture also showed the growth of mucormycosis species. Antifungal therapy in the form of amphotericin was initiated, and right lobectomy was performed. The resected specimen measured 15 × 10 × 4 cm, and the upper pole showed a 5 ×5 × 3 cm circumscribed necrosed area. Histological examination showed necrotic tissue containing plenty of sparsely septate, broad-based, thick-walled hyaline fungal hyphae along with mixed inflammatory infiltrate and a few foreign body giant cells. Adjacent lung parenchyma also showed inflammatory consolidation with similar fungal profiles (**a** HE ×400, **b** PAS ×400 and **c** FNAC HE ×400)

Mucormycosis Renal Allograft

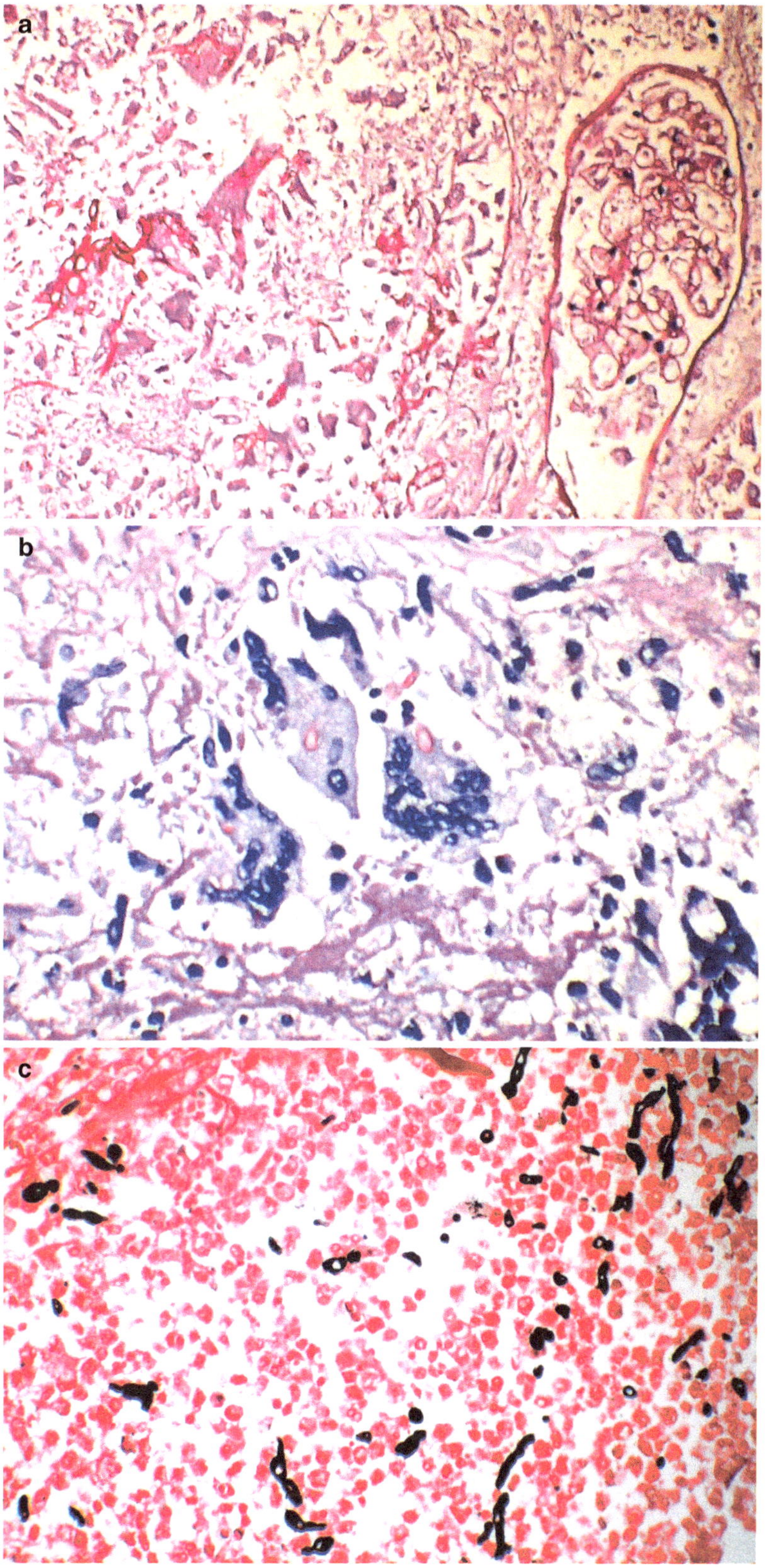

Fig. 4.44 (**a**–**c**) A 55-year-old male received live-related renal allograft about 3 years ago. He was maintained on triple drug immunosuppression. He presented with drop in urine output for 2 months. Ultrasonographic examination revealed markedly swollen and enlarged graft with complete loss of corticomedullary details. Renal Doppler of the graft kidney showed decreased renal parenchymal vascularization. Lab workup revealed hemoglobin 5.8 g/dl and TLC 21000/cu mm with 83 % neutrophils; platelets were 111000/cu mm. Serum Cr 4.6 mg/dl and BUN 61 mg/dl. Soon the patient developed advanced renal failure, and graft nephrectomy had to be performed. Intraoperatively, the graft kidney was found soft, flaccid, and ruptured. Gross examination of explanted renal allograft showed multiple subcapsular infarcts with areas of hemorrhage and necrosis. Microscopic examination showed wide areas of hemorrhagic necrosis infiltrated with irregular, broad, and aseptate fungal hyphae having wide-angle branching and prominent angioinvasion. The fungal elements were also seen inside the giant cells. The diagnosis of zygomycosis was offered (**a** HE ×400, **b** PAS ×400 and **c** CSM ×400)

Mucormycosis Colon in a Renal Allograft Recipient

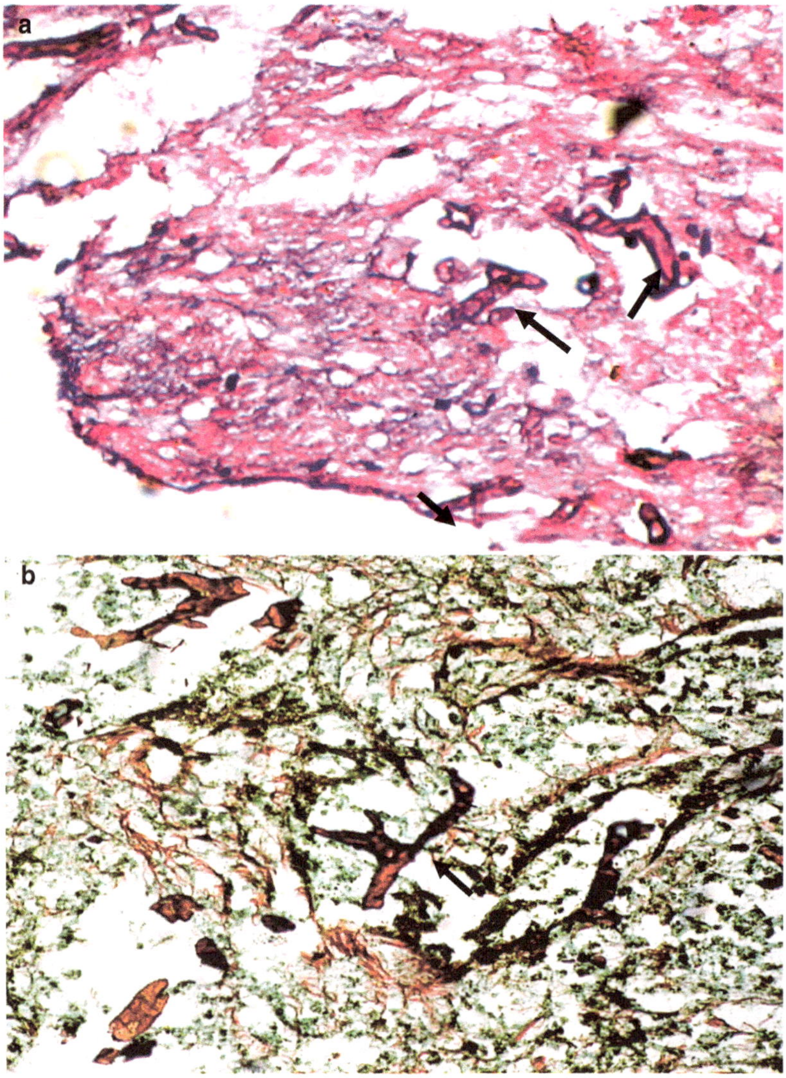

Fig. 4.45 (**a**, **b**) A 37-year-old male renal allograft recipient on triple drug immunosuppression, 6 months post-transplant presented with acute abdomen. The abdomen was tense and tender. X-ray of the abdomen showed multiple fluid levels. Emergency laparotomy revealed colonic perforation. Biopsy from the site of perforation showed necrotic tissue infiltrated with multiple broad aseptate thick-walled irregular fungal hyphae (*arrows*), suggestive of mucormycosis (**a** HE ×400 and **b** CSM ×400)

Mucormycosis of the Liver in an HIV-Positive Patient

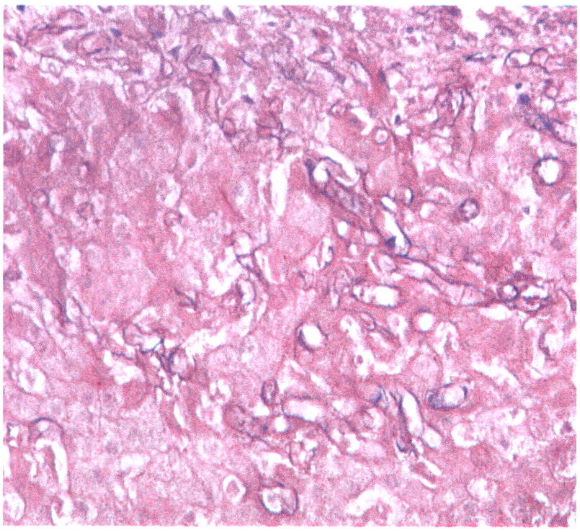

Fig. 4.46 A 50-year-old male patient presented with diffuse abdominal pain and distension. He had the history of repeated commercial sexual exposures and was found to be HIV positive. The patient died within 48 h after hospitalization. Autopsy showed gastric perforation with peritonitis. The liver was 1100 g, and cut surface shows several necrotic areas. Microscopic examination revealed mild periportal inflammatory infiltrate consisting of mixed population of neutrophils and lymphocytes against necrotic background. The liver parenchyma was necrotic showing fair number of broad, irregular, and aseptate fungal hyphae suggestive of mucormycosis (HE ×400) (Contributor – Dr. Anjali Amrapurkar, Department of Pathology, KLM Hospital, Mumbai, India)

Orbital Mucormycosis in a Diabetic Patient

Fig. 4.47 (**a–g**) A 60-year-old male patient known to have been suffering with uncontrolled diabetes mellitus for 7 years along with chronic renal failure presented with moderate fever for 20 days and hemoptysis and epistaxis for 8 days. He also had right-sided facial weakness. On the basis of CT and laboratory workup, he was diagnosed to have rhinocerebral mucormycosis. Right-sided orbital exenteration was performed. Postoperative recovery was uneventful; however, the patient died on the 3rd postoperative day due to cardiopulmonary arrest. Histopathological examination of the exenterated eyeball along with attached optic nerve and periorbital tissue showed mixed inflammatory infiltrate with confluent areas of aseptic necrosis along with broad, aseptate, irregular, and thick-walled fungal hyphae invading the periorbital tissue, optic nerve, and the retina (*arrows*); angioinvasion was also seen. A diagnosis of mucormycosis of the orbit was offered (**a** HE ×200, **b–d** PAS ×200, **e** PAS ×400, **f**, **g** CSM ×400)

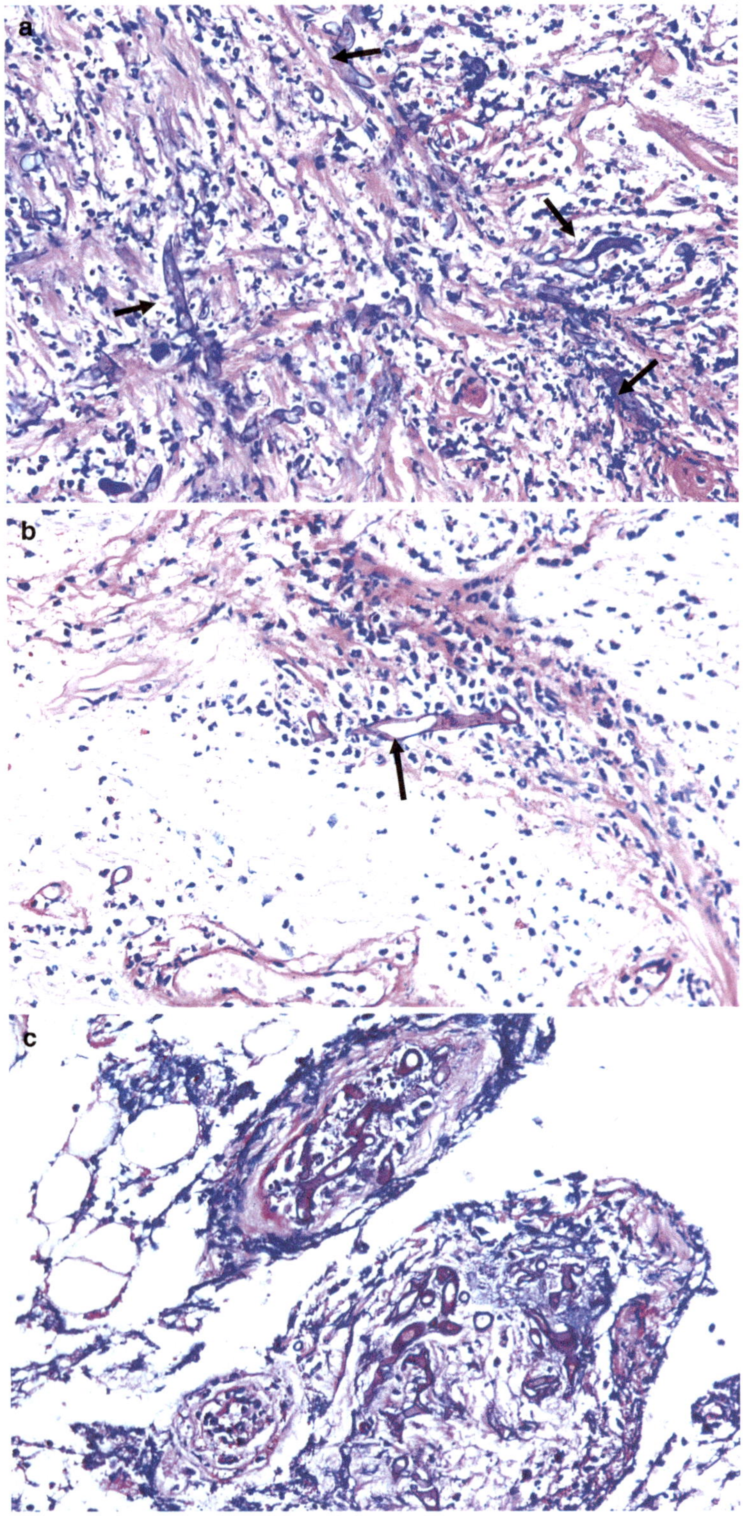

Fig. 4.47 (continued)

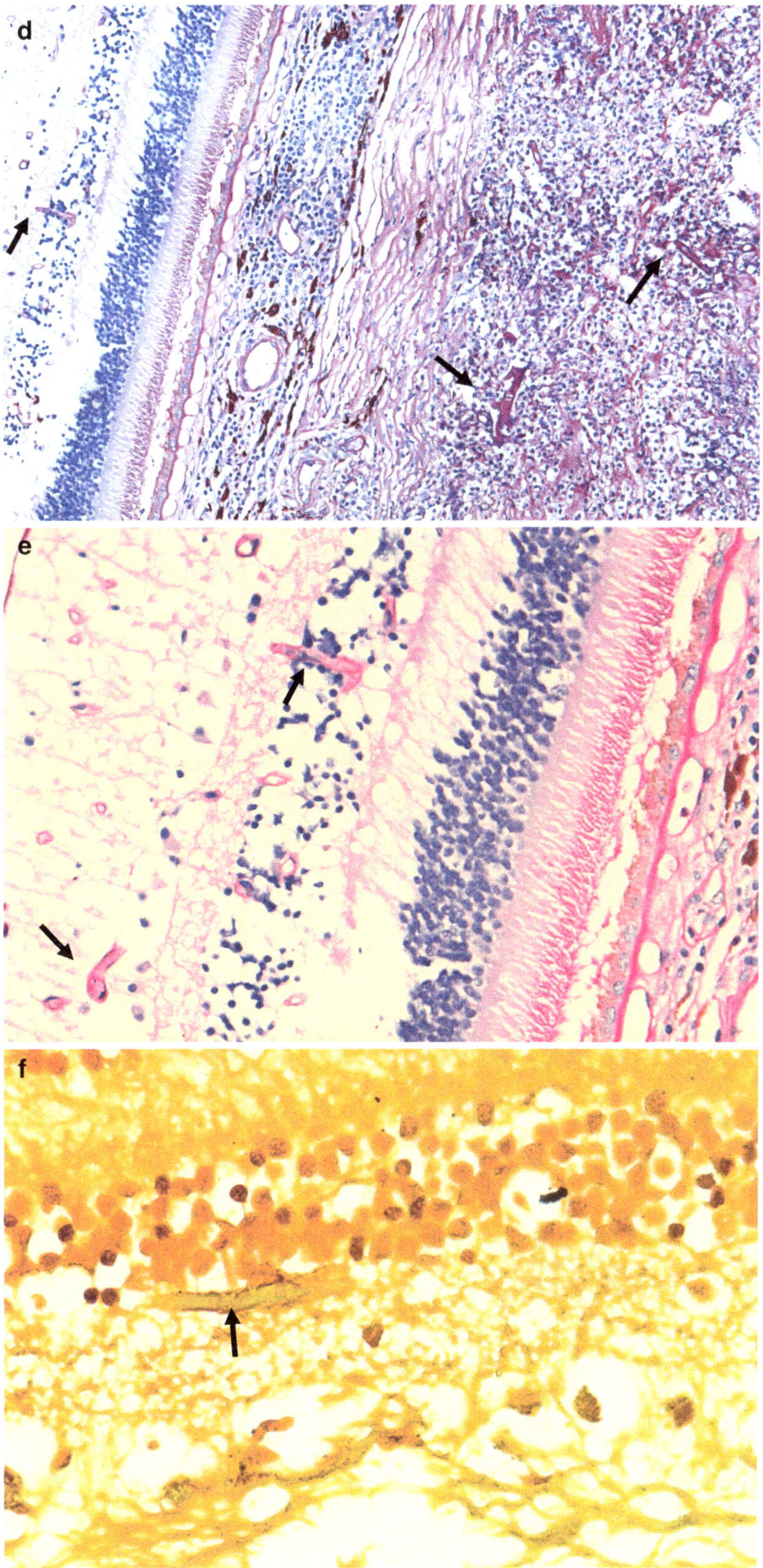

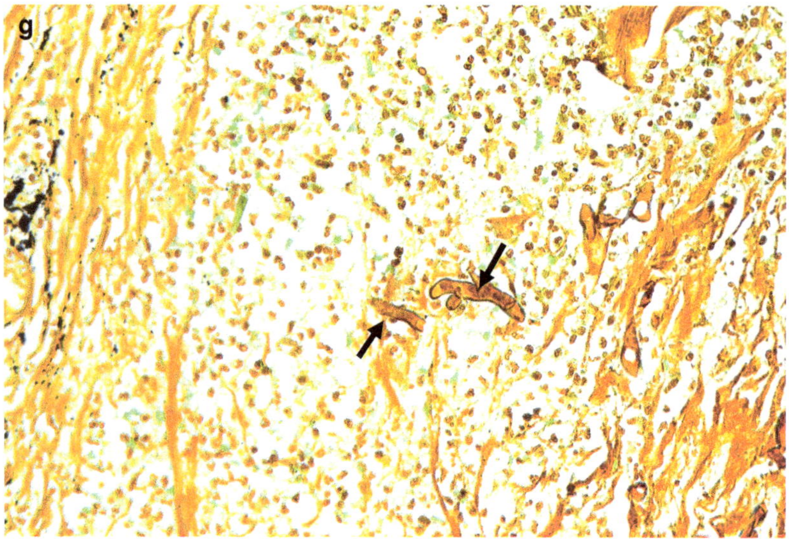

Fig. 4.47 (continued)

Mucormycosis of the Brain in a Diabetic Patient

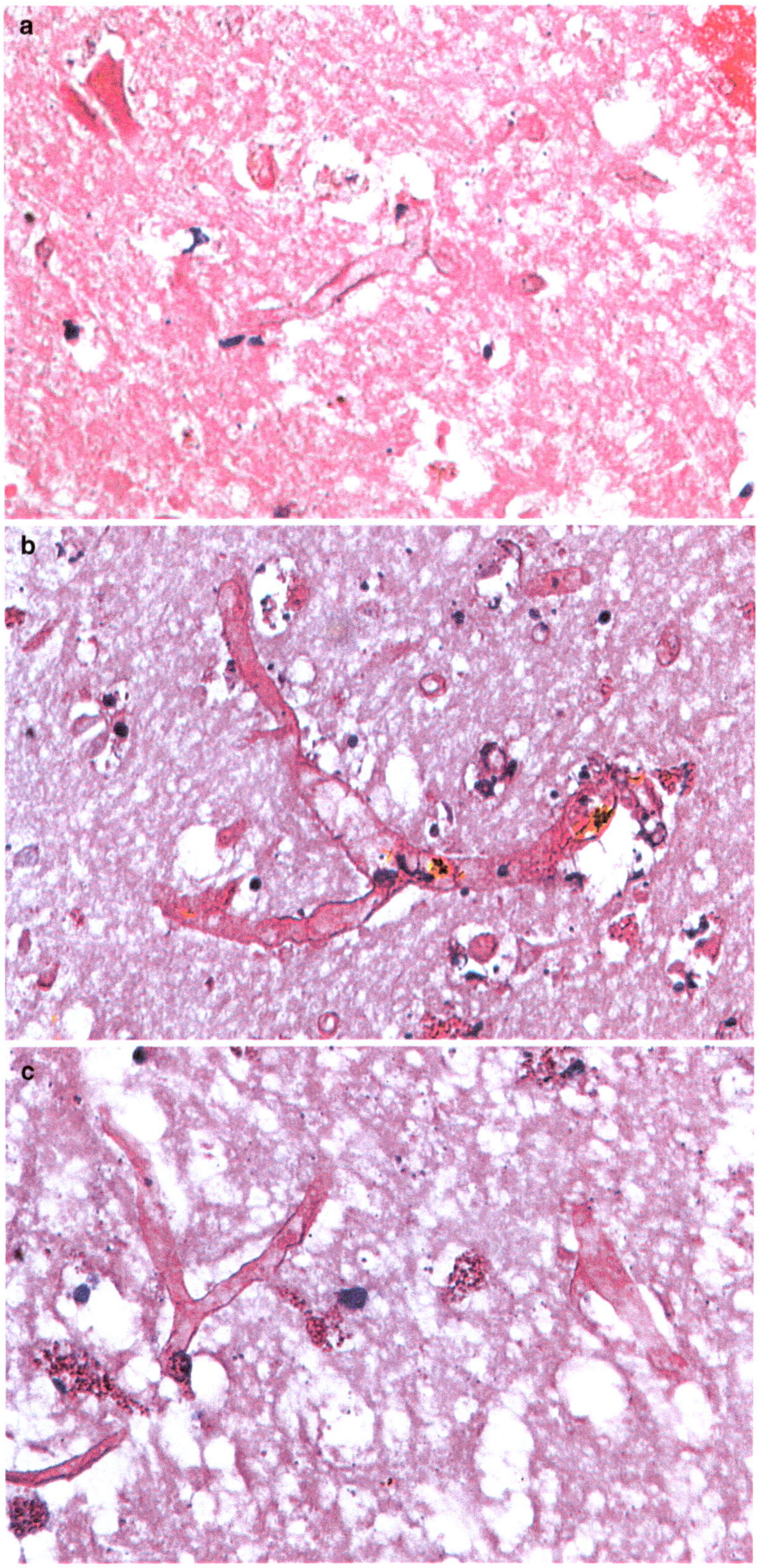

Fig. 4.48 (**a**–**c**) A 65-year-old male patient presented with mild to moderate holocranial headache for 1 month followed by sudden onset speech arrest and weakness of the right upper and lower limbs for 20 days. Clinical examination revealed loss of muscle power in both the right upper and lower limbs (1/5); however, there was no sensory or cranial nerve deficit. Laboratory workup revealed that the patient was diabetic with RBS of 232 mg/dl; blood counts revealed TLC 8740/cu mm with 70 % polys. Viral markers were negative. At surgery, brain parenchyma was found necrosed. Histological examination showed broad irregular thick-walled irregularly branched aseptate fungal profiles suggestive of mucor infiltrating brain parenchyma (**a** HE ×200, **b**, **c** PAS ×400)

Phaeohyphomycosis (Dematiaceous Molds): The dematiaceous molds are characterized by the presence of brown or black color in the cell wall. The fungus occurs as saprophyte in soil and decaying organic matter. Phaeohyphomycosis may clinically manifest as superficial, cutaneous, or subcutaneous infection or as mycotic keratitis. At times, invasive or systemic disease presenting as cerebral abscess may also be encountered; it has rapidly declining clinical course.

In tissue sections, the fungus shows dark brown elongated conidiophores producing branched acropetal chains of smooth-walled conidia. PAS and GSM stain the fungus well; Masson-Fontana stain for melanin stains the fungus black. The determination of etiological agent of phaeohyphomycosis needs identification by culture.

Differential diagnosis includes chromomycosis which also appears brown in tissue section but shows thick-walled muriform or sclerotic bodies, which are divided by septation.

Phaeohyphomycosis: Ulcer Knee in a Renal Allograft Recipient Developing Posttransplant Diabetes Mellitus (PTDM)

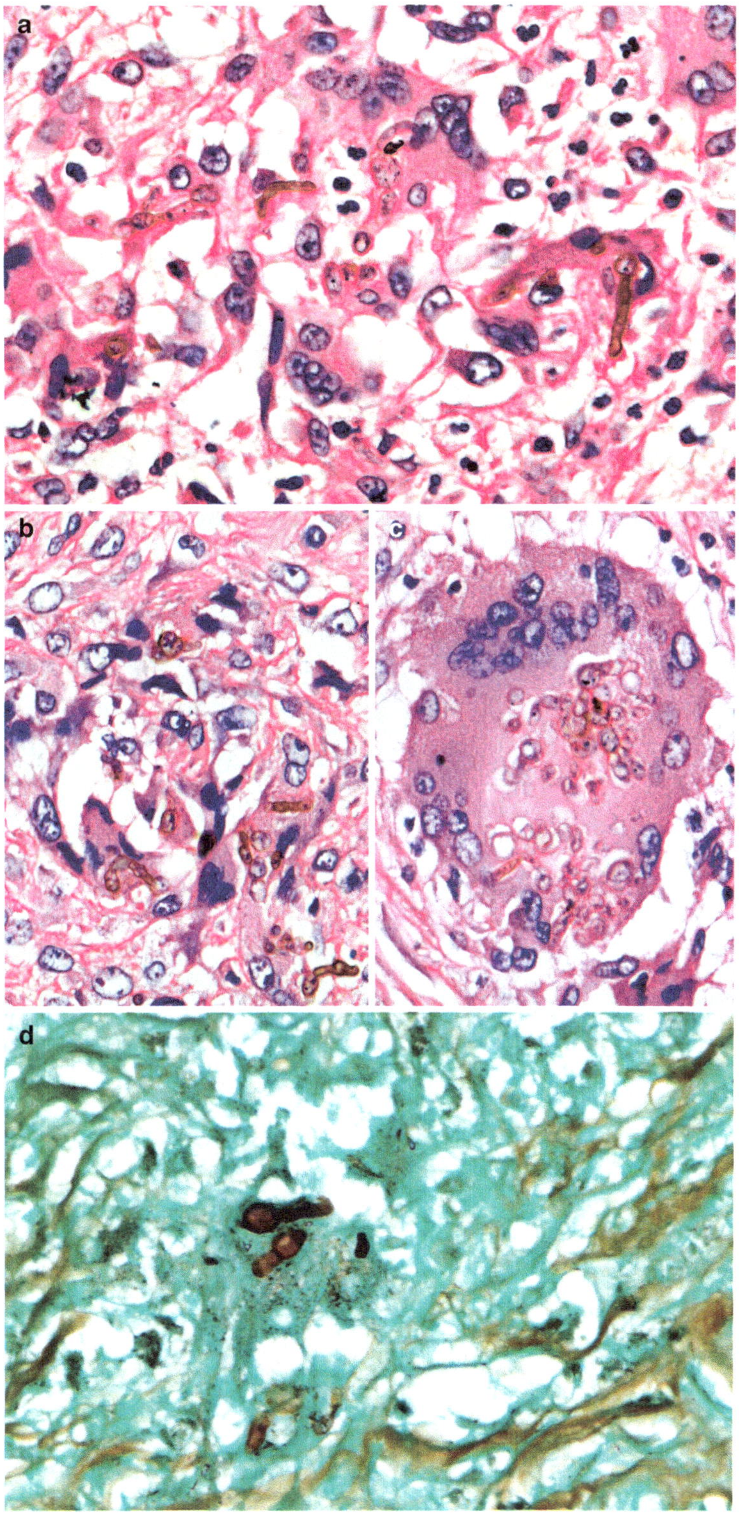

Fig. 4.49 (**a–d**) A 31-year-old male patient receiving live-related renal allograft developed posttransplant diabetes mellitus; 3 years posttransplant, he presented with a nonhealing ulcer with multiple discharging sinuses on the right knee joint for 3 months. The excision of the ulcer was done. The histopathological examination showed brown-colored broad irregular pseudo hyphae and partially septate hyphae of phaeohyphomycosis both within and outside the giant cells (**a–c** HE ×200 and **d** CSM ×400)

Phaeohyphomycosis: Hand Swelling in a Patient with Diabetic Nephropathy on Hemodialysis

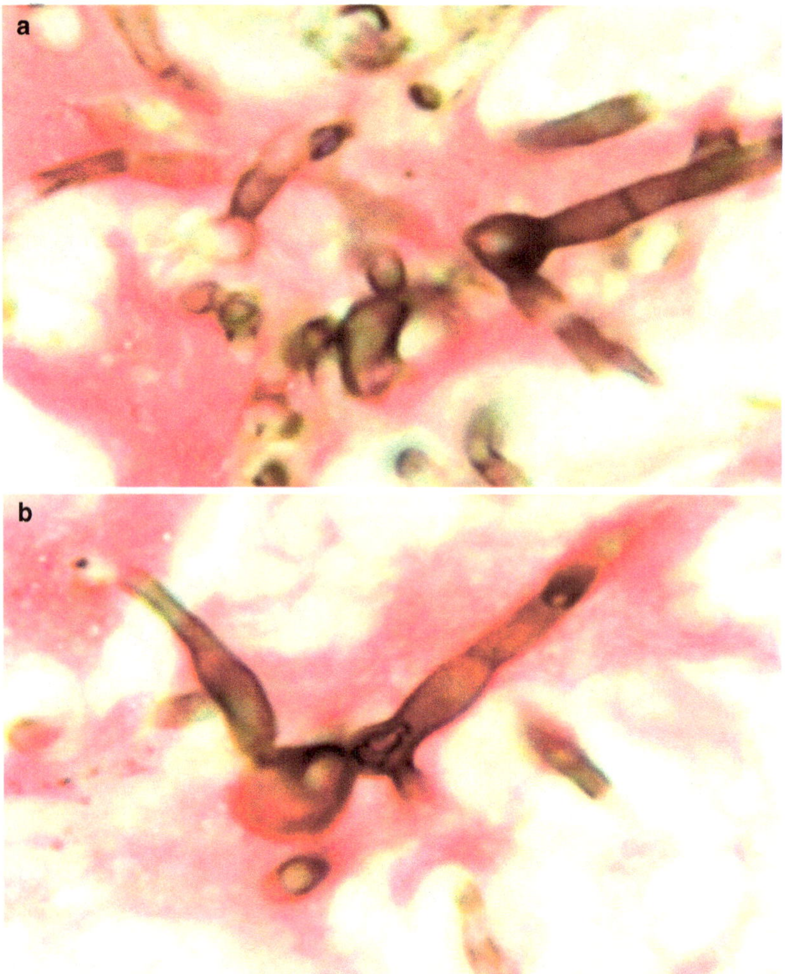

Fig. 4.50 (**a**, **b**) A 53-year-old male patient who was diabetic for 15 years presented with renal failure and was on hemodialysis. He developed swelling on the dorsum of the hand for 10 days; the swelling was nontender, 1.5 × 1.0 cm in size, and freely mobile. Biopsy of the swelling revealed broad, pseudo hyphae, and partially septate brown-colored hyphae of phaeohyphomycosis (**a**, **b** HE ×400) (Contributor – Dr. S Radha, Kamineni Hospital, Hyderabad, India)

Phaeohyphomycosis of the Brain in a Renal Allograft Recipient

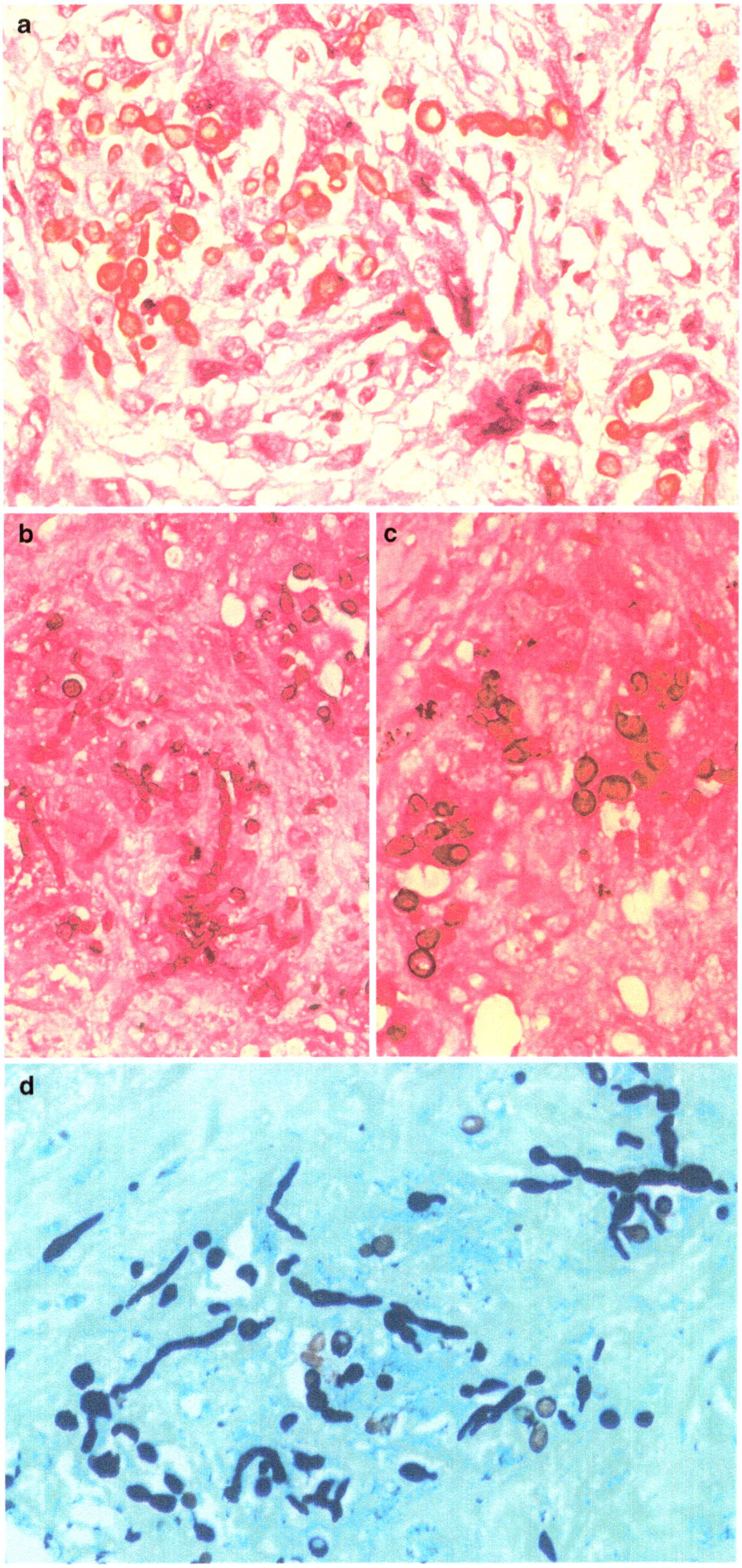

Fig. 4.51 (**a**–**g**) A 56-year-old male patient who received live-related renal allograft a year ago and was being maintained on triple drug immunosuppression and presented with altered sensorium and vomiting for 10 days. MRI revealed an irregular necrotic SOL in the right parietal lobe with conglomeration of multiple nodular and ring-enhancing lesions surrounding it, involving the right thalamus and extending to the frontotemporal lobe up to the subependymal region. Craniotomy was performed and the histopathological examination of the excised tissue revealed necrotic brain parenchyma diffusely infiltrated with *dark brown* elongated conidiophores producing branched acropetal chains of smooth-walled conidia yeastlike cells, septate hyphae, and pseudo hyphae along with rounded thick-walled conidia of phaeohyphomycosis (**a** HE ×400, **b**, **c** PAS ×400 and **d** CSM ×400, **e** Masson-Fontana ×400). Culture on Sabouraud's dextrose agar revealed slowly growing, *dark olive black*, compact fungal colonies; the microscopic examination showed elongated conidiophores producing branched acropetal chains of smooth-walled conidia, and based on the morphological features, the fungus was identified as *Cladosporium carrionii* (**f**, **g** Lactophenol cotton *blue* ×400) (Contributor to mycological workup – Dr. Vipul Kumar Srivastava, Consultant Microbiologist, Sahara Hospital, Lucknow, India)

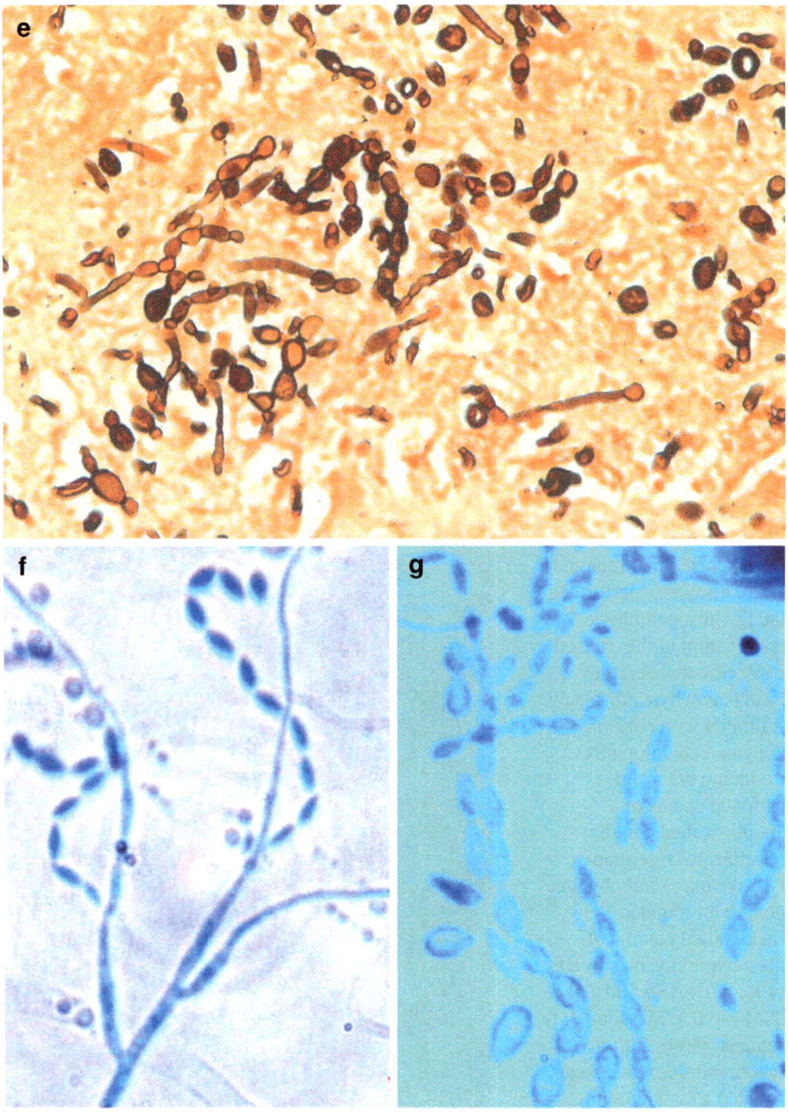

Fig. 4.51 (continued)

Fusarium: *Fusarium* species are widely distributed as natural flora in soil, decaying plant material, and other organic debris and water. *Fusarium* spp. are important plant pathogens. However, occasionally animals and man can also be infected. *Fusarium* can be identified by the production of hyaline banana-shaped multicellular macroconidia and hyaline globose and smooth- to rough-walled chlamydoconidia.

Depending on host immune status, *Fusarium* sp. cause wide spectrum of infections in humans. Superficial (keratitis and onychomycosis) and localized (wound infection) disease occurs mostly in immunocompetent patients. Although *Fusarium* has not been identified as opportunistic fungal pathogen, it, however, causes invasive and disseminated disease in immunocompromised patients. The important risk factor for severe fusarosis includes prolonged neutropenia and T-cell immunodeficiency. The prognosis in these patients is poor and is determined largely by the degree of immunosuppression and extent of infection, with almost 100 % mortality among persistently neutropenic patients.

Fusarium: Postoperative Wound Infection

Fig. 4.52 (**a–f**) A 45-year-old male patient underwent surgery for prolapsed intervertebral disk (PIVD). Thereafter, he developed wound infection at the operated site which did not respond to antibiotics. The granulation tissue from the wound was removed; the histopathological examination showed chronic granulation tissue with foreign body giant cell reaction along with hyaline banana-shaped multicellular macroconidia and hyaline globose and smooth- to rough-walled chlamydoconidia of *Fusarium*; at places fungal elements were also seen within the giant cells (*arrows*). Slide culture for fungus showed hyaline, branched septate hyphae bearing hyaline banana-shaped microconidia in clumps on monophialides and occasional three-celled macroconidia (*arrow*), characteristic of *Fusarium* sp. (**a–c** HE ×400, **d** CSM ×400, **e**, **f** Lactophenol cotton *blue* ×400) (Contributor to mycological workup – Dr. Vipul Kumar Srivastava, Consultant Microbiologist, Sahara Hospital, Lucknow, India)

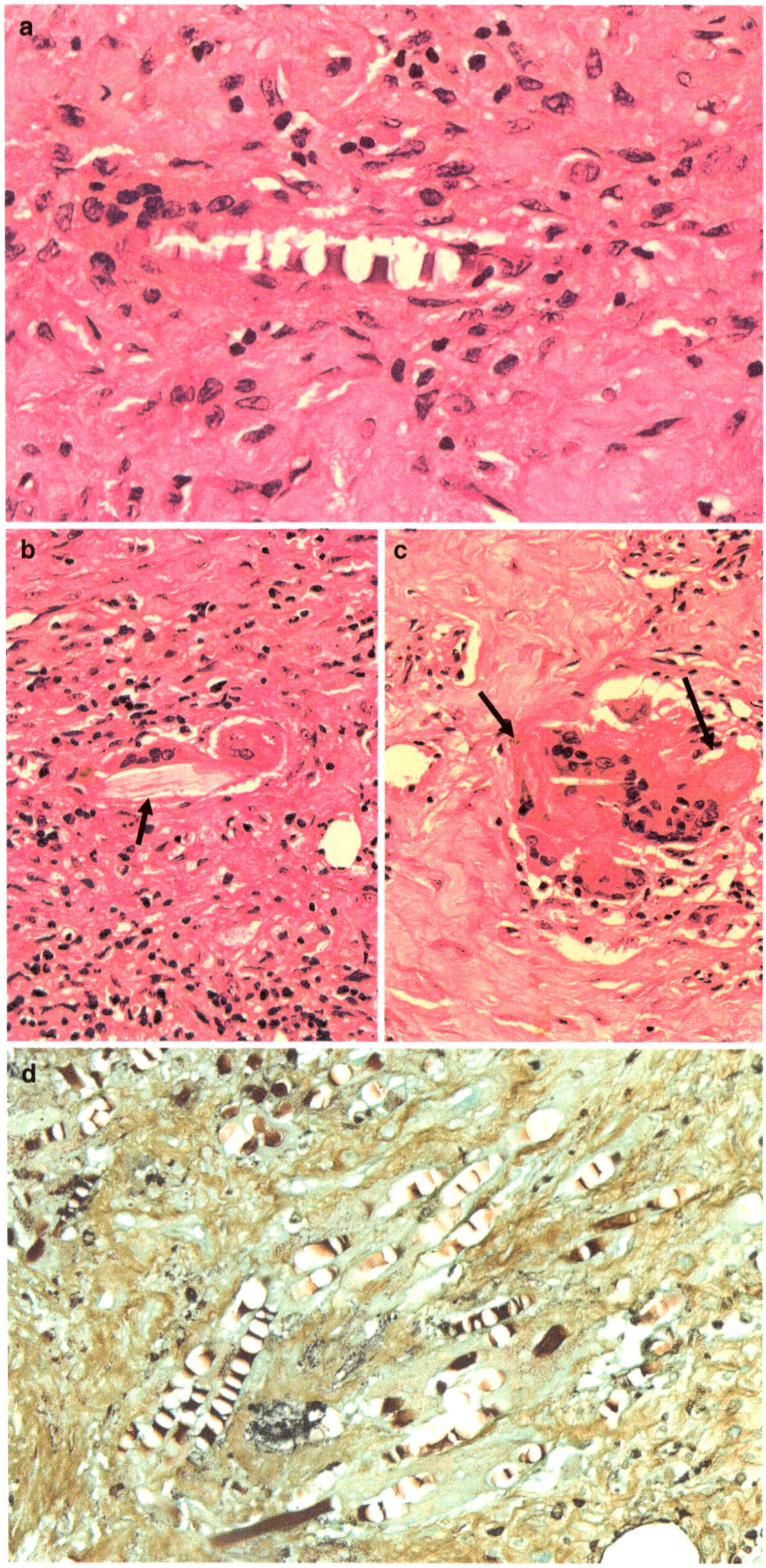

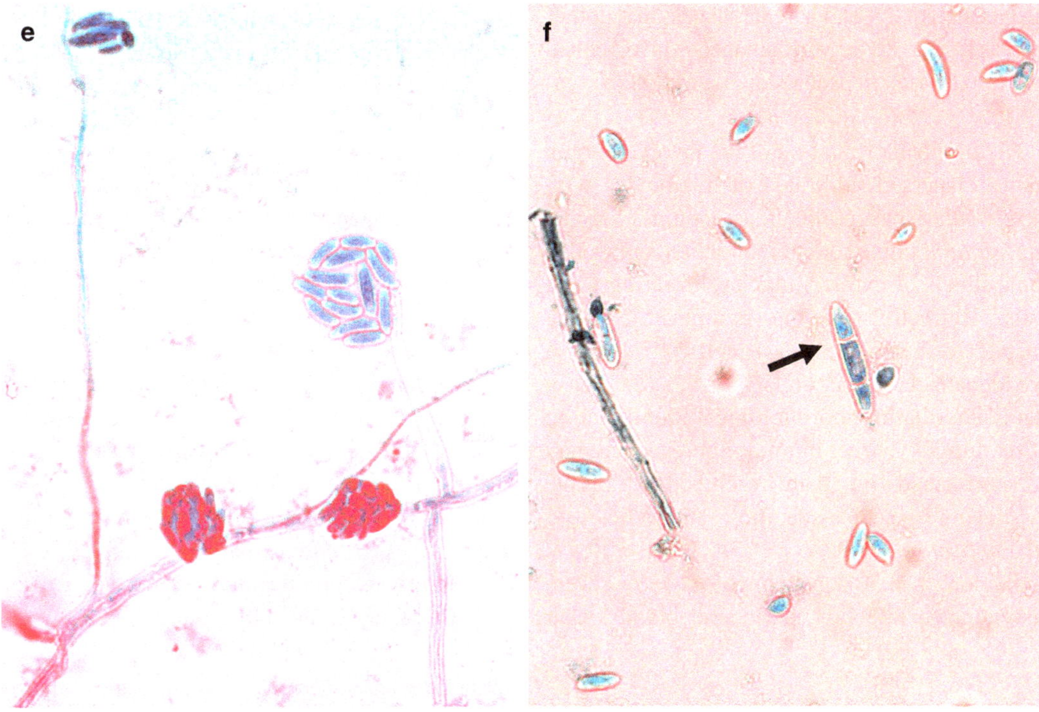

Fig. 4.52 (continued)

Histoplasma: *Histoplasma* are dimorphic fungi, the myecelial form is infective. Two variants, viz., *H. capsulatum* var capsulatum and *H. capsulatum* var duboisii, are pathogenic.

Histoplasma capsulatum **(Causative Agent of Classical Histoplasmosis, Small-Cell Histoplasmosis, Darling's Disease, Cave Disease, Spelunker's Disease):** Immunocompromised individuals are prone to develop systemic fungal infection by *H. capsulatum*; HIV-infected patients usually develop histoplasmosis when CD4 counts are <200/ul. The infection is acquired by inhalation. Lungs are the primary site of involvement; 5–10% patients may present with disseminated disease. Dissemination occurs by hematogenous route involving bone marrow, pericardium, mediastinum, GIT, and adrenal glands; the mortality is as high as 80 %. Mucocutaneous involvement may also be seen in patients of HIV/AIDS.

Histological evaluation of the involved organ shows dispersed infiltrates of histiocytes with intracellular basophilic blastoconidia of *H. capsulatum*; immunodeficient patients may also show sheets of extracellular proliferating yeast cells. Retraction of the cytoplasm of the phagocyte from the yeast cells produces a pseudocapsular effect on HE, PAS, and Giemsa stains, facilitating morphological identification of the fungus. Direct immunofluorescence may be performed on paraffin-embedded tissue by using species-specific antibodies to *Histoplasma*.

In more than 50 % patients of AIDS or severe disseminated infection, peripheral blood smear may show yeast-laden macrophages. The organisms can also be demonstrated on bronchoalveolar lavage or fine-needle aspirate smears.

Besides, culture, techniques like complement fixation, agar gel diffusion, radioimmunoassay, PCR, and specific oligonucleotide probes can be used for antigen detection in early cases. Rapid identification in culture can be done by exoantigen test or the chemiluminescence labeled DNA probe.

Histoplasma duboisii **(Causative Agent of African Histoplasmosis, Large Cell Histoplasmosis):** *H. duboisii*-induced skin lesions manifest as papules and noduloulcerative lesions. Osseous lesions show osteolysis. In tissue biopsies, *H. duboisii* appear as large (10–15 um), lightly basophilic thick-walled yeast cells with a profound giant cell reaction.

Table 4.4 Major differences in clinical features between *H. capsulatum* and *H. duboisii*

Organs involved	*H. capsulatum*	*H. duboisii*
Lung	More common	Less common
Skin and bone	Less common	More common

From: Gupta RK. In *Pathology of opportunistic infections in tropics*. Jaypee; 2007

Histoplasma Liver in an Immunocompromised Patient

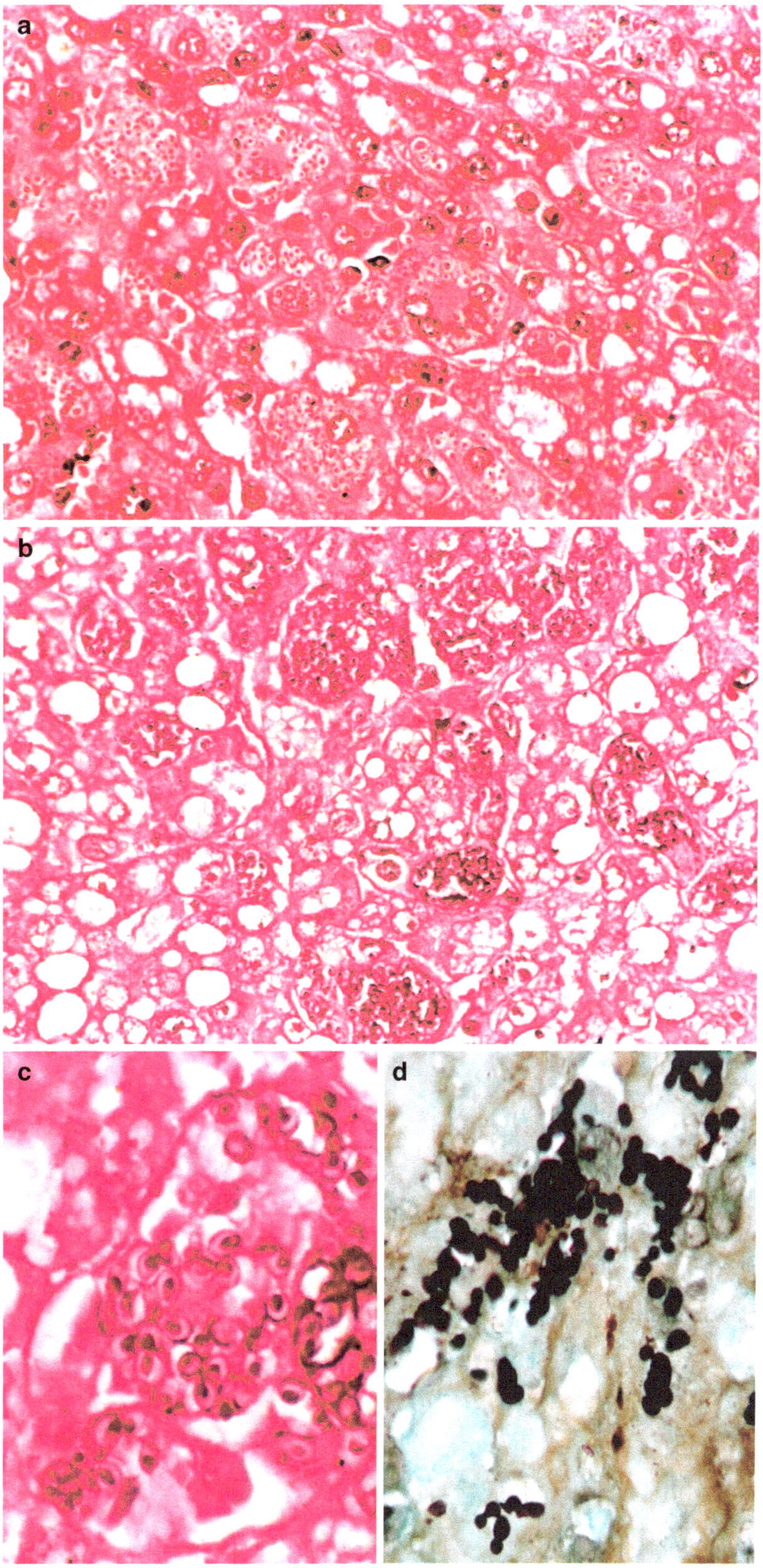

Fig. 4.53 (**a**–**d**) A 25-year-old female patient known to have been suffering from dermatomyositis was on prolonged immunosuppressant therapy. She presented with septicemia and hepatomegaly and died within 72 h after hospitalization. Postmortem liver biopsy showed extensive infiltration of Kupffer cells by *Histoplasma*; parenchymal granulomas studied with *Histoplasma* were also seen (**a** HE ×400, **b** PAS ×400, **c** PAS ×1000 and **d** Masson-Fontana ×1000)

Histoplasma of the Tongue After Radiotherapy for Tongue Squamous Cell Carcinoma

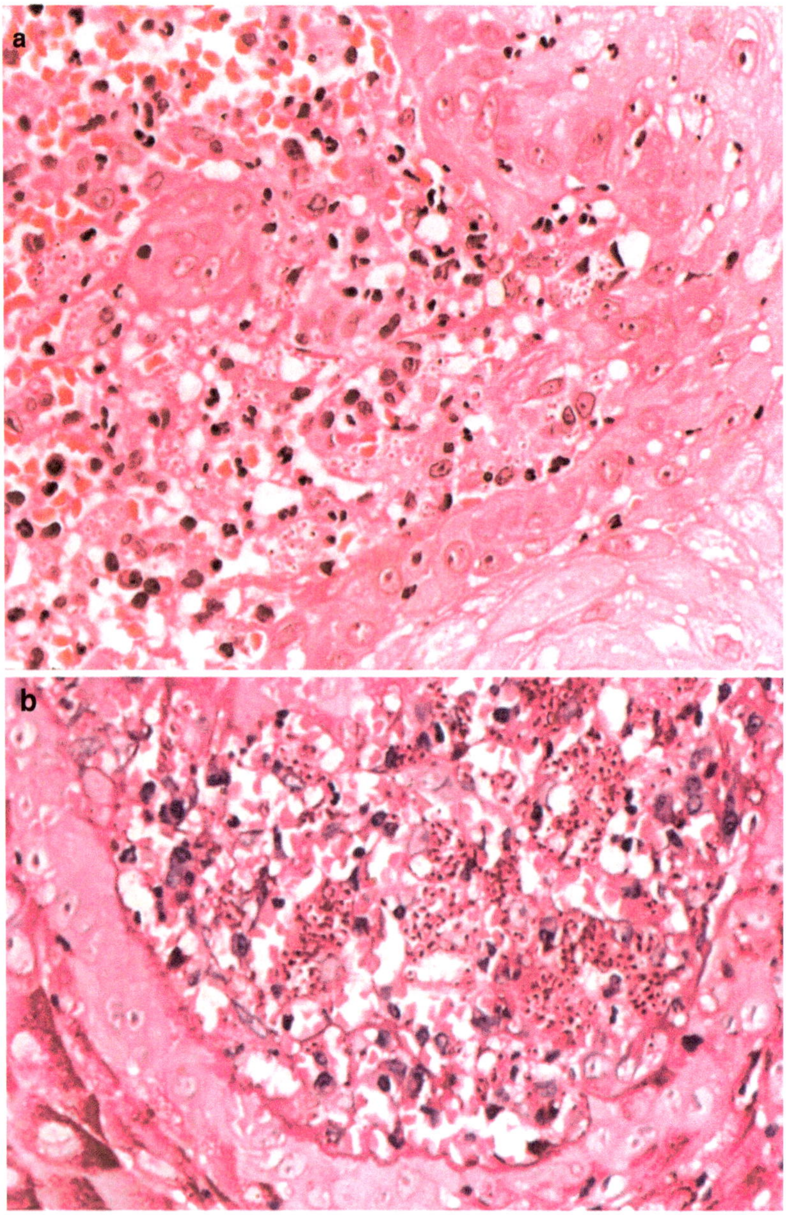

Fig. 4.54 (**a**–**b**) A 55-year-old male patient, who was receiving radiotherapy for keratinizing squamous cell carcinoma of the tongue, during postradiotherapy phase presented with a nonhealing ulcer on the tongue. Biopsy from the ulcer showed the presence of *Histoplasma* within histiocytes (**a** HE ×400, **b** PAS ×400) (From: Gupta RK. In *Pathology of opportunistic infections in tropics*. Jaypee; 2007)

Histoplasmosis of Adrenals (Bilateral) in a Patient with Pulmonary Tuberculosis

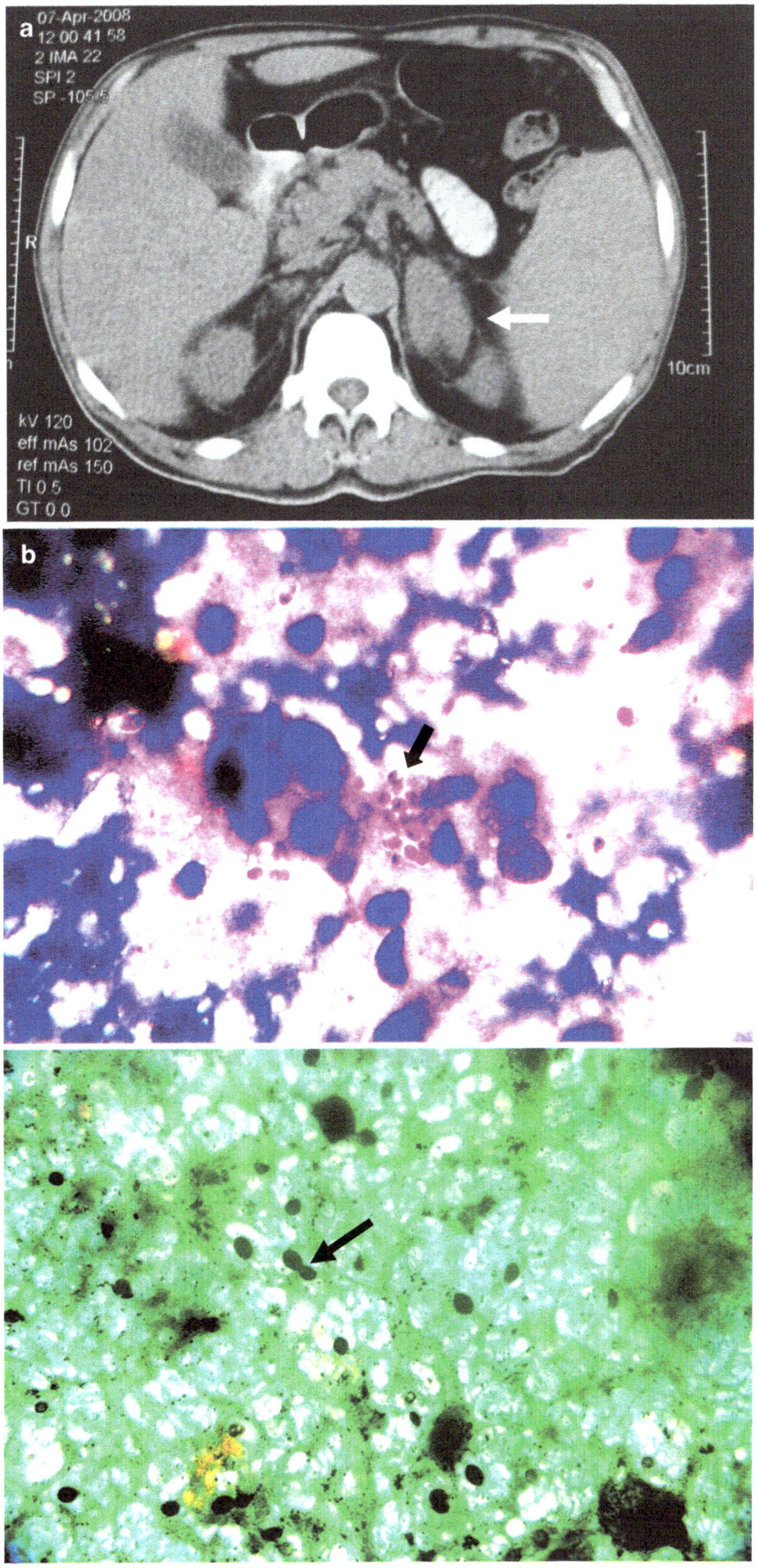

Fig. 4.55 (**a**–**e**) A 48-year-old male patient who was on ATT for pulmonary tuberculosis presented with fever, weight loss, increasing weakness, and progressive generalized pigmentation all over the body for 10 months. Physical examination revealed hepatomegaly (3 cm) and splenomegaly (2 cm). Routine laboratory parameters were within normal limits. Abdominal CT showed bilateral enlargement of adrenals, each measuring 6 cm in size (**a**). CT-guided FNAC from the adrenals showed multiple capsulated yeastlike organisms suggestive of *Histoplasma* (**b** MGG ×400, **c** CSM ×400, **d** Masson-Fontana ×400). Histopathological examination of the resected adrenal also showed plenty full intracellular and extracellular capsulated yeastlike organisms of *Histoplasma* (**e** HE ×400)

Fig. 4.55 (continued)

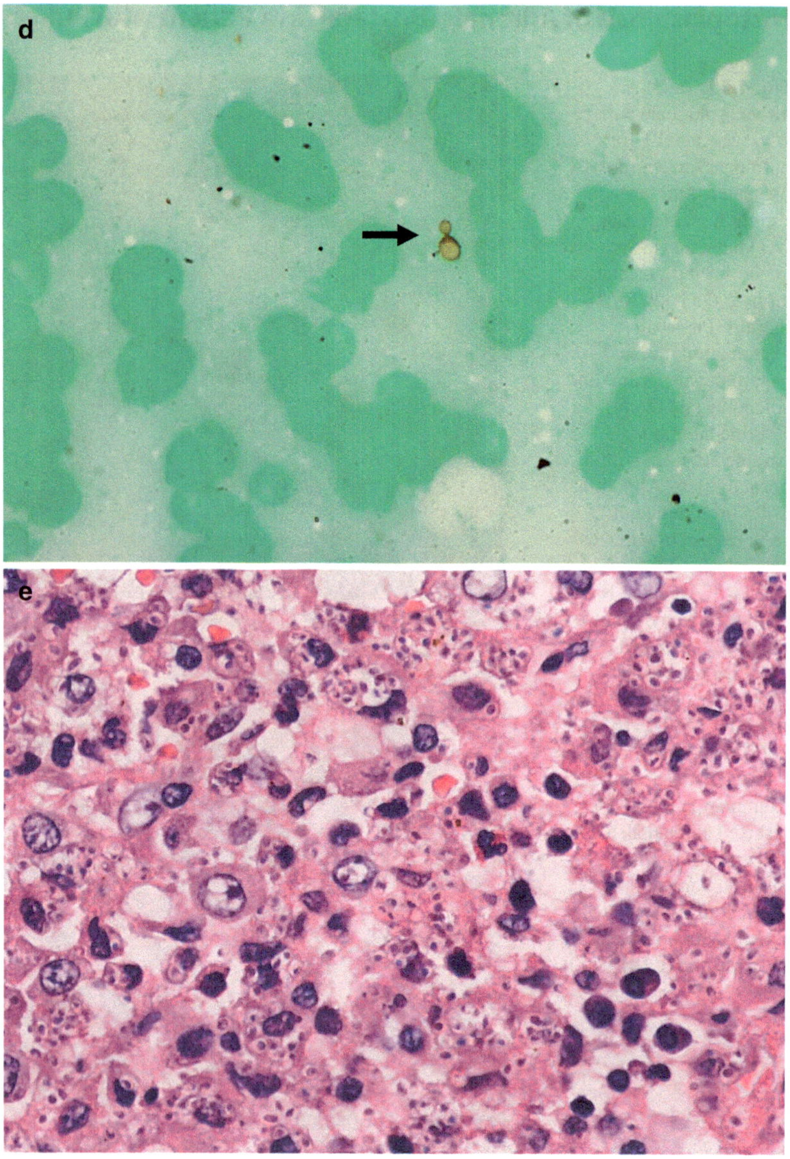

Histoplasma in Bone Marrow and Lymph Node in a Patient with Pancytopenia

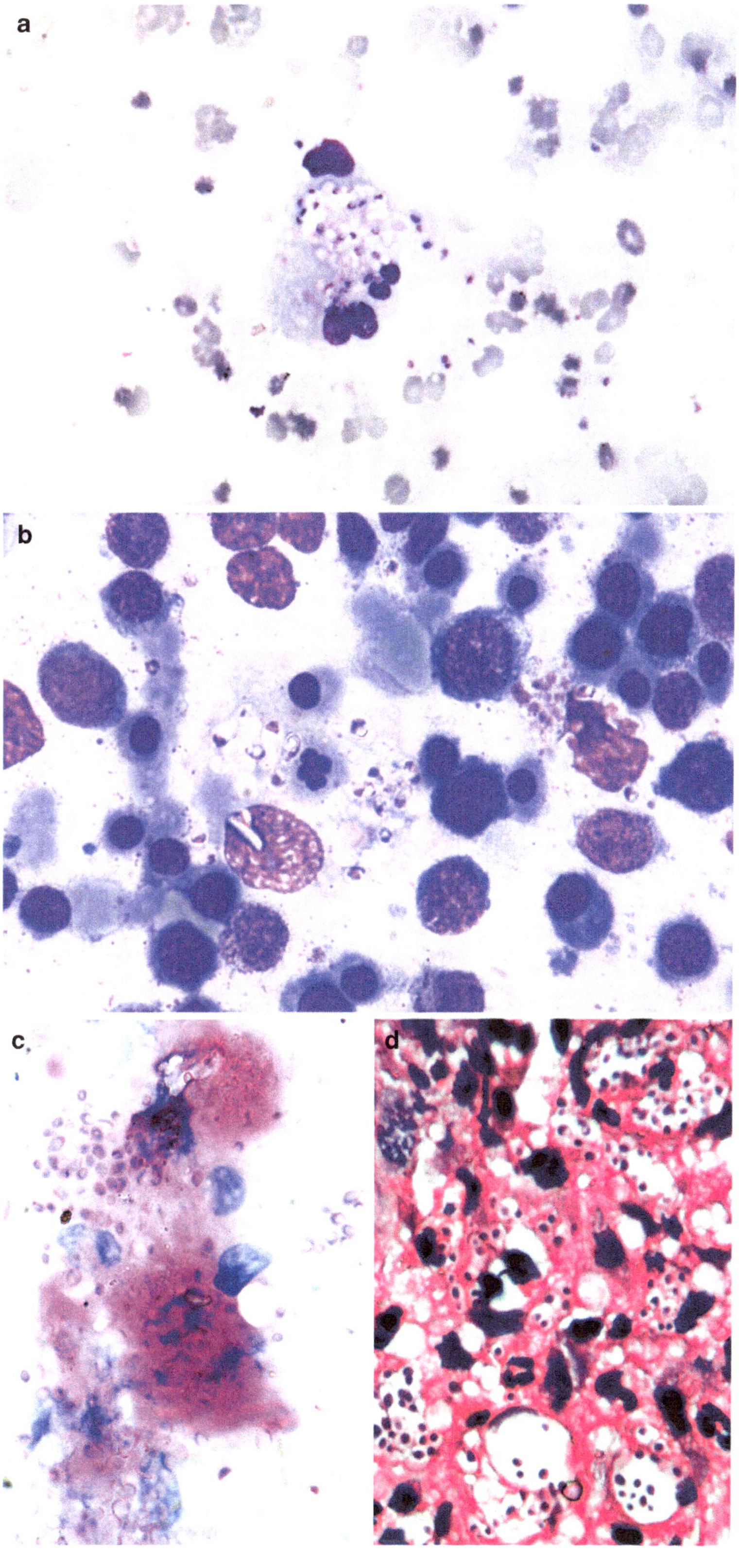

Fig. 4.56 (**a**–**d**) A 25-year-old male patient presented with persistent high-grade fever associated with marked weight loss for 2 months and abdominal pain for 15 days. Investigations revealed pancytopenia and abdominal lymphadenopathy. Bone marrow aspirate showed increased number of macrophages with intracytoplasmic fungal yeasts of *Histoplasma capsulatum* (**a** Leishman ×400, **b** Leishman ×1000). Lymph node aspirate smears (**c** PAS ×1000) and lymph node biopsy also showed similar PAS-positive fungal elements (**d** PAS ×1000)

Histoplasmosis of the Skin and Lung in a Patient with Wegener's Disease

Fig. 4.57 (**a–g**) A 30-year-old female, a known case of Wegener's granulomatosis on steroids and cyclophosphamide since 5 months, presented with fever and dry cough for 2 months. CT of the thorax showed multiple nodular lesions in both lungs; there was no lymphadenopathy. She had erythematous dusky papular lesions on both arms and face. Lab investigations revealed hemoglobin 7.1 g/dl, total WBC count 13,000/cu mm, Ser creatinine 1.2 mg/dl, and C-ANCA 60 U/ml. Punch biopsy from the skin lesion showed presence of fair number of yeastlike capsulated organisms suggestive of *Histoplasma* (**a** HE ×200, **b** CSM ×400). Lung biopsy also showed similar organisms (**c** HE ×200, **d** CSM ×400). The kidney biopsy showed crescentic glomerulonephritis with the presence of noncaseating epithelioid granuloma in periglomerular area; a medium-sized artery with reduplication of internal elastic lamina is also seen (**e** HE ×200, **f**, **g**. PAS ×200)

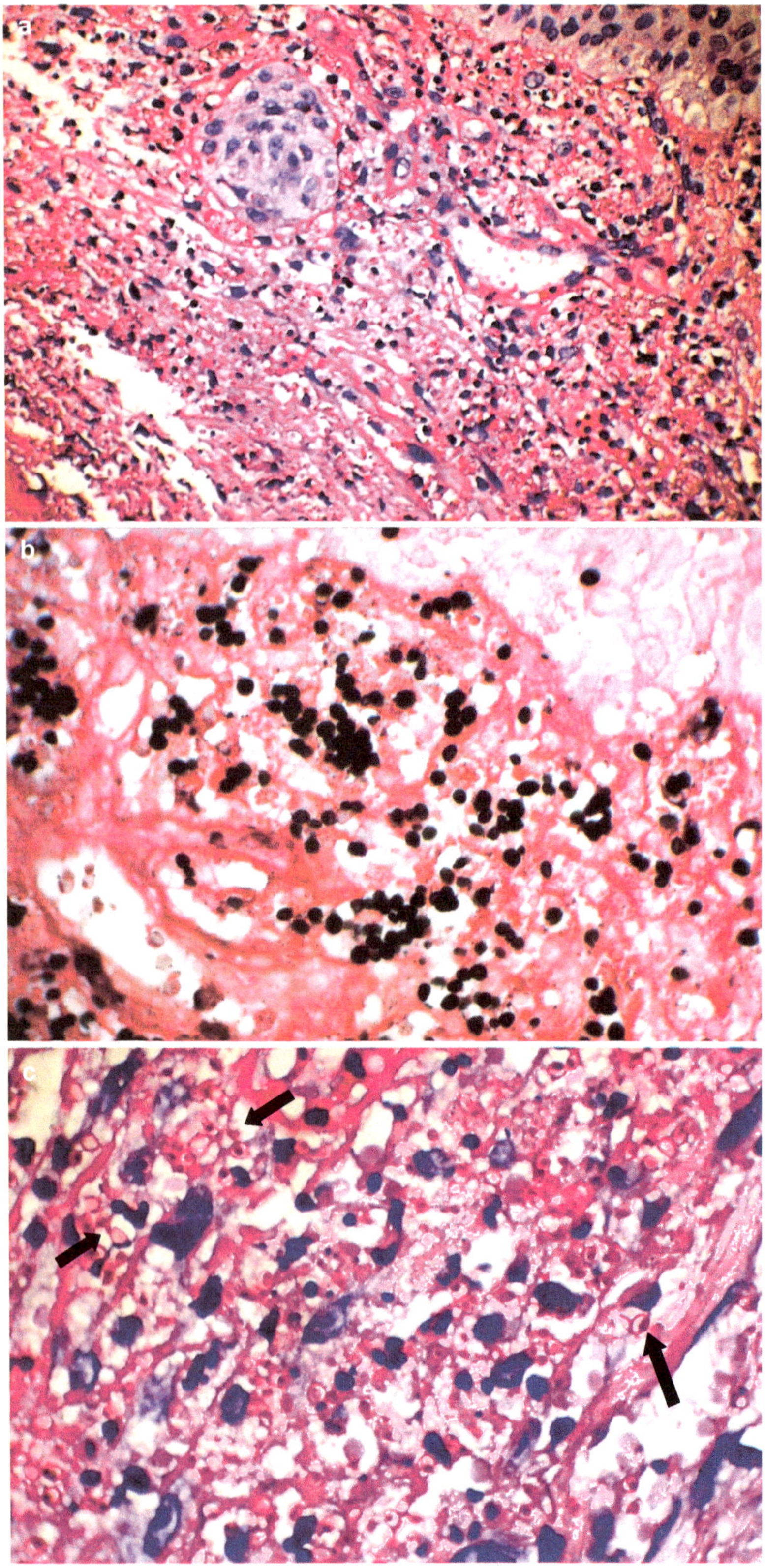

Fig. 4.57 (continued)

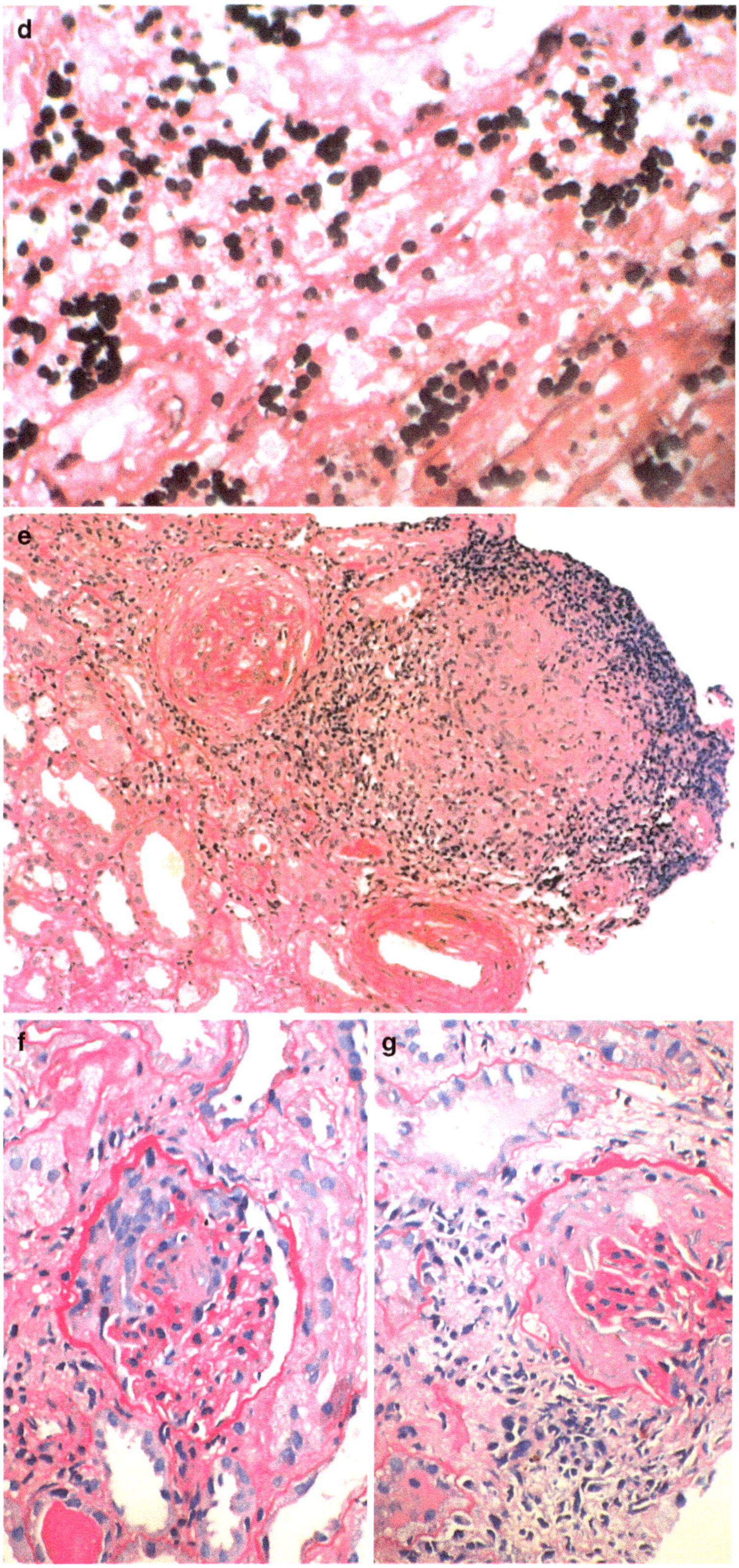

Histoplasma of the Cecum in an Immunocompromised Patient (A Case of Disseminated Histoplasmosis)

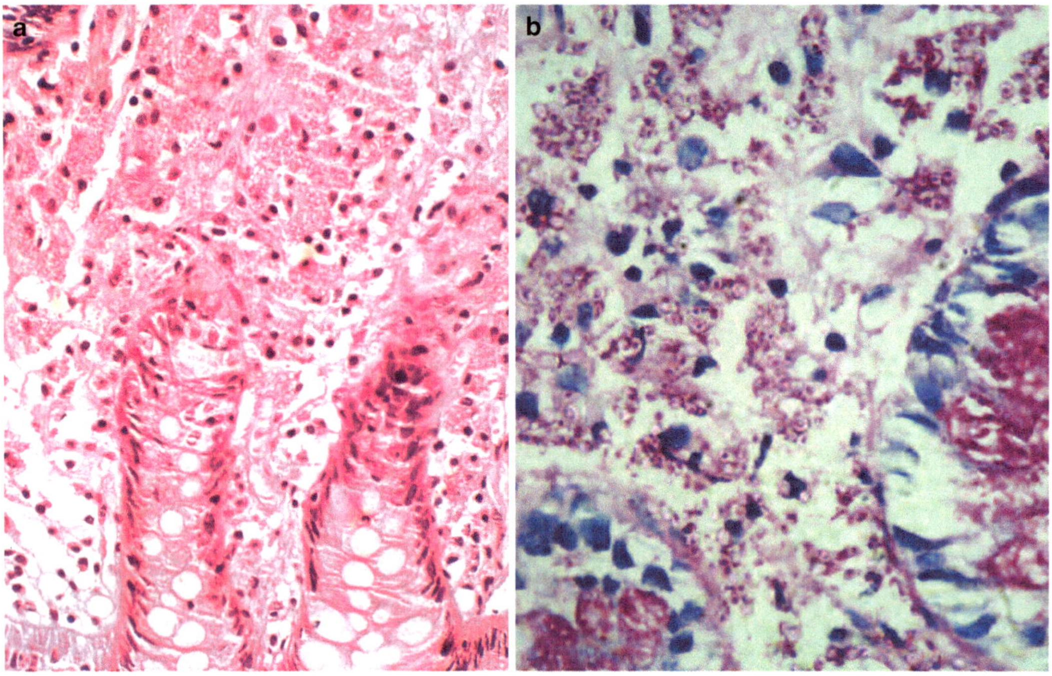

Fig. 4.58 (**a**, **b**) A 55-year-old male patient, known to have HBV-related cirrhosis, presented with low-grade fever, constipation, and off and on colicky abdominal pain for 6 months along with oral ulceration and recent onset of lower GI bleed. Lower GI endoscopy revealed loss of vascular pattern in the colon. Biopsy from the cecum and colon showed *Histoplasma*. Examination of sputum and oral ulcer scrape smears also showed the presence of similar yeastlike organisms suggestive of disseminated histoplasmosis (**a** HE ×400 – negative shadows and **b** PAS ×1000) (From: Gupta RK. In *Pathology of opportunistic infections in tropics*. Jaypee; 2007)

Disseminated Histoplasmosis

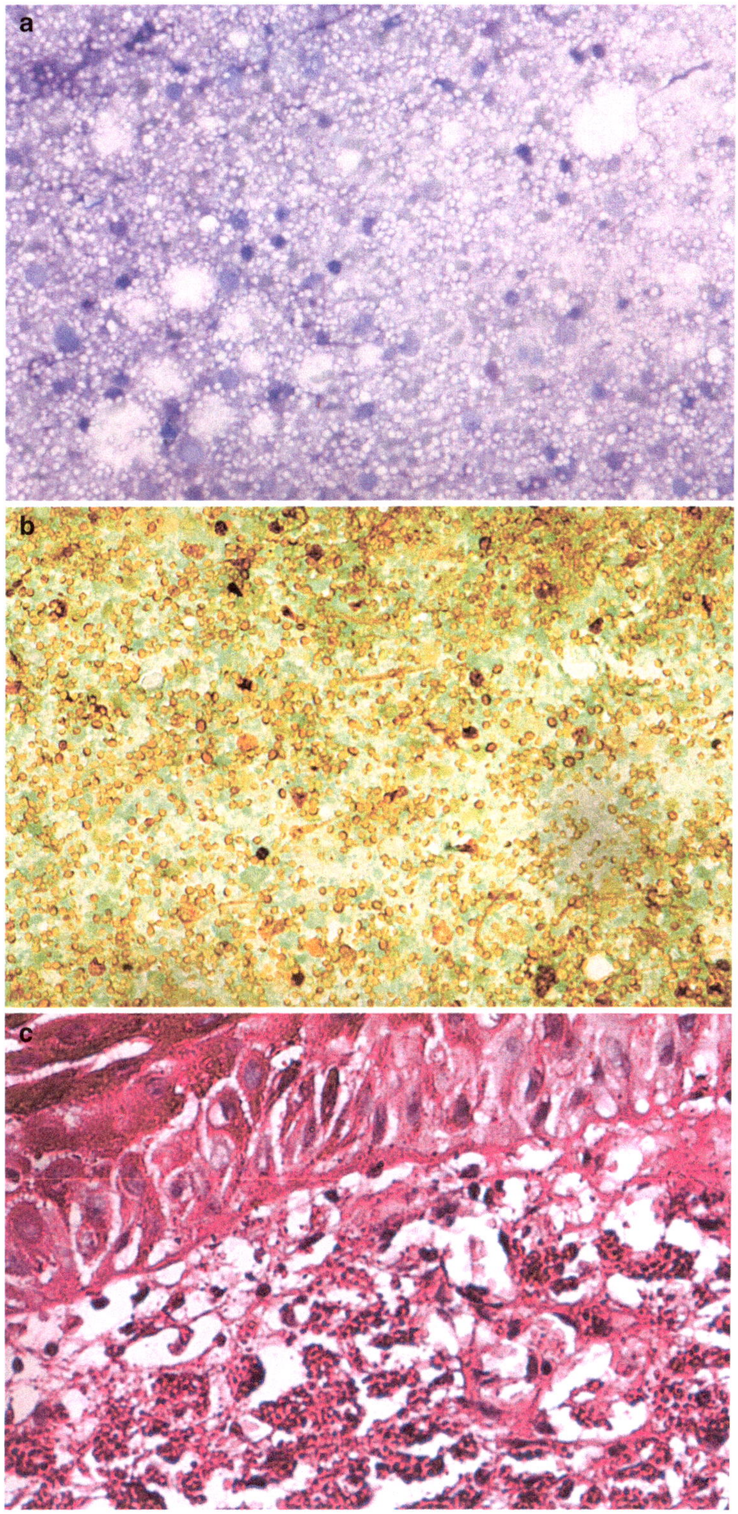

Fig. 4.59 (**a**–**f**) A 60-year-old female patient presented with h/o low-grade intermittent fever and weight loss for 6 months (received prolonged course of multiple antibiotics). Subsequently during the last 4 months, she developed multiple painless nodular skin lesions particularly on the flexure aspect of the elbow, eyelids, abdominal wall, and trunk. Past history was not relevant. On examination, she was found to have bilateral enlarged jugulodigastric lymph nodes which were hard and nontender. She also had multiple whitish elevated or nodular oral lesions on gingival and buccal mucosa and hard palate. Multiple fleshy nontender skin nodules on the flexure aspect of the elbow, eyelids, abdominal wall, and trunk, waxy in consistency, were also present. Liver was enlarged 2 cm below the right subcostal margin in midclavicular line; it was firm and nontender. The spleen was also enlarged 4 cm below the left subcostal margin; it was firm and nontender. Any skeletal lesions were not identified. USG of the abdomen revealed hepatosplenomegaly. Chest X-Ray PA was WNL. Laboratory investigations revealed pancytopenia along with raised ESR (110 mm/ Westergreen). Fasting blood sugar was 126/dl. Serology for ANA and HIV was negative, and the routine urine examination was WNL. FNA cervical LN (**a** MGG ×400 – negative shadows, **b** CSM ×400), Skin biopsy (**c** PAS ×400, **d** Masson-Fontana ×400), bone marrow aspiration (**e** PAS ×400), and FNAC from adrenal (**f** PAS ×400) showed large number of yeastlike capsulated fungal elements suggestive of disseminated histoplasmosis

Fig. 4.59 (continued)

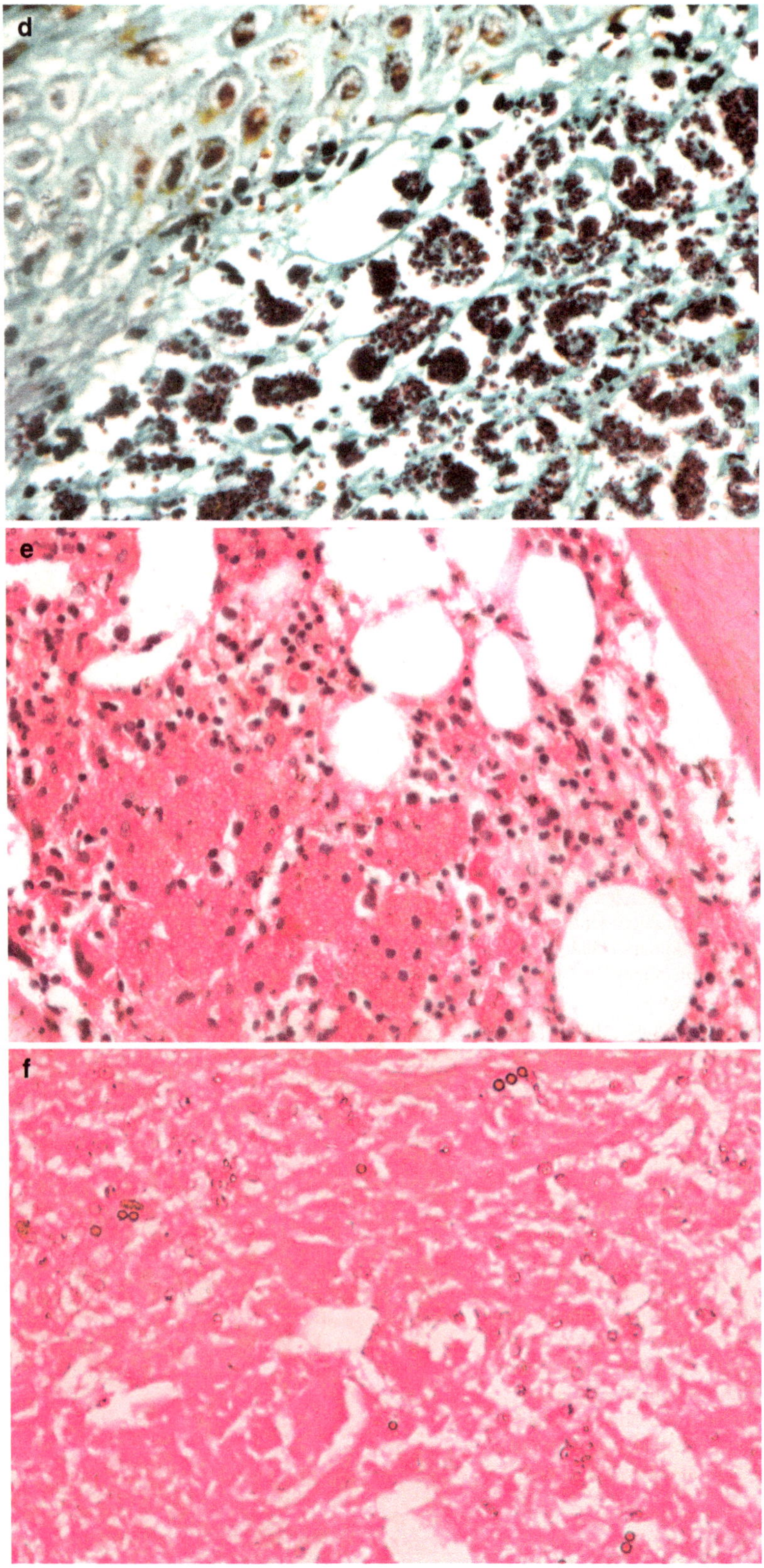

Further Reading

1. Agarwal V, Gupta RK, Jain M. Invasive fungal infections is renal allograft recipients. Indian J Pathol Microbiol. 2005;48:448–52.
2. Ajello L. Hyalohyphomycosis and phaeohyphomycosis: two global disease entities of public health importance. Eur J Epidemiol. 1986;2:243–51.
3. Banerjee SN, Ewori TG, Culven DH, et al. Secular trends in nosocomial primary bloodstream infections in the United States. 1980–89. Am J Med. 1991;91:863–95.
4. Bodey GP. Gametogenous and major organ candidiasis. In: Bodey GP, editor. Candidiasis: pathogenesis, diagnosis and treatment. 2nd ed. New York: Raven Press; 1993. p. 279–329.
5. Butha BJ, Bensett SR, Johnson AC. Disseminated inoculation blastomycosis in a renal transplant recipient. Am Rev Respr Dis. 1984;130:1180.
6. CDS. Control and prevention. CDC surveillance summaries, surveillance for AIDS-defining opportunistic illnesses. 1992–1997. Morb Mortal Wkly Rep. 1999;48(no. 22–2):1–22.
7. Chandler FW, Watts JC. In: Connor DH, Chandler FW, editors. Pathology of infectious diseases. Stamford: Appleton & Lange; 1997. p. 991.
8. Chandler FW, Kaplan W, Ajello L. Histopathology of mycotic diseases. Chicago: Year Book Medical Publishers; 1980.
9. Chandler FW, Watts JC. Phaehypnopycosis. In: Connor DH, Chandler FW Schwartz DA, Manz HJ, Lack EE, editors. Pathology of infectious diseases. Stamford: Appleton & Lange; 1997. pg 1060.
10. DCD Recommend for prophylaxis against Pneumocystis carinii pneumonia for adults and adolescents infected with HIV. MMWR. 1992;41:1–11.
11. Deng Z, Connor DH. Progressive disseminated penicilliosis caused by Penicillium marneffei: report on eight cases and differentiation of the causative organism from histoplasma capsulatum. Am J Clin Pathol. 1985;84:323–7.
12. Drouhet E and Dupont B. Candidiasis in heroin addicts and AIDS: new immunology data on chronic mucocutaneous candidiasis. In: Candida and candidiasis. New York: Plenum Press; 1991. p. 61–72.
13. Edman JC, Kovacks JA, Masur H, et al. Ribosomal RNA sequence shows pneumocystis carinii to be a member of the fungi. Nature. 1998;334:519–22.
14. Eras P, Goldstem MJ, Shirlock P. Candida infection of the GI tract. Medicine. 1972;51:367–79.
15. Fish DG, Anpel NM, Galniani JN, et al. Coccidioidomycosis. Showing human immunodeficiency virus infection: a review of 77 patients. Medicine. 1990;69:384–91.
16. Fishman JA, Rubin RH. Infections in organ transplant recipients. N Engl J Med. 1998;338:1741–51.
17. Frater JL, Hall GS, Procop GW. Histologic features of zygomycosis: emphasis on perineural invasion and fungal morphology. Arch Pathol Lab Med. 2001;125:375–8.
18. Galgiani JN. Coccidioidomycosis: a regional disease of national importance. Rethinking approaches for control. Ann Intern Med. 1999;130:293–300.
19. Gilchrist TC, Stokes WR. A case of pseudo-lupus vulgaris. Caused by a Blastomyces. J Exp Med. 2013;3:53–78.
20. Goodrich JM, Reed EC, Mori M, et al. Clinical features and analysis of risk factors for invasive candidal infection after marrow transplantation. J Infect Dis. 1991;164:731–40.
21. Grimley PM, Wright CD, Jennings AE. Torulopsis glabrata infection in man. Am J Clin Pathol. 1965;43:216–23.
22. Gupta RK, Jain M, Garg R. Pneumocystis carinii pneumonia after renal transplantation. Indian J Pathol Microbiol. 2004;47:474–6.
23. Gupta RK. Opportunistic infections in renal allograft recipients. Transplant Proc. 2007;39:731–3.
24. Gupta RK. Opportunistic fungal infections. In: Pathology of opportunistic infections in tropics. New Delhi: Jaypee; 2007. p. 35.
25. Hazer KC, Howell SA. Candida, cryptococcosis other yeasts of medical importance. In: Murray PR, editor. Manual of clinical microbiology. Washington, DC: Oxford Journals; 2007.
26. Hemochowicz S, Sahovic E, Pistole M, et al. Histoplasmosis diagnosed on peripheral blood smear from a patient with AIDS. JAMA. 1985;253:3148.
27. Jha S, Ghosh P, Agarwal V. Cryptococcal meningitis unmasking idiopathic CD4 lymphocytopenia. Neurol India. 2007;55:312–4.
28. Kerkering TM, Duma RJ, Shadomy S. The evaluation of pulmonary cryptococcosis: clinical implications from a study of 41 pts. With & without compromising host factors. Ann Intern Med. 1981;94:611–6.
29. Khalil MA, Hassan AW, Gugnani HC. African histoplasmosis: report of four cases from North Eastern Nigeria. Mycoses. 1998;41:293–5.
30. Lee CH, Lan RS, Tsai YH, et al. Riv's stain in the diagnosis of pulmonary Cryptococcosis: introduction of a new diagnostic method. Chest. 1988;93:467–70.
31. Maksymiuk AW, Thonsprasert S, Hobfer R, Luna MA, Fainstcin V, Bodey GP. Systemic candidiasis in cancer patients. Am J Med. 1984;77:20–7.
32. Marina NM, Flynn PM, Rivera GK, Hughis WT. Candida tropicalis and candida albicans fungaemia in children with leukaemia. Cancer. 1991;68:594–9.
33. Marks MI, Langston C, Epekhoff TC. Torulopsis glabrata – an opportunistic pathogen of man. N Engl J Med. 1970;283:1131–5.
34. Mc Ginnis MR. Chromoblastomycosis and phaeohyphomycosis: new concepts, diagnosis and mycology. J Am Acad Dermatol. 1983;8:1–15.
35. Mills J. Pneumocystis carinii and Toxoplasma gondii infections in patients with AIDS. Rev Infect Dis. 1986;8:1001–11.
36. Mitchell TG, Perfect JR. Cryptococcosis in the era of AIDS – 100 years after the discovery of C. neoformans. Clin Microbiol Rev. 1995;8:515–48.

37. Myerowitz RL. Localized and disseminated candidiasis. In: Myerowitz RL, editor. The pathology of opportunistic infections. New York: Raven Press; 1983. p. 95–114.
38. Ng VL, Yajko DM, Hadley WK. Extrapulmonary pneumocystosis. Clin Microbiol Rev. 1997;10:401–18.
39. Nolan MT, Long JP, Mac Rean DP, Mxfitzge G. Aspergillosis and lung fibrosis. B J Med Sci. 1985;154:336–42.
40. Nucci M, Anaissie E. Fusarium infection in immunocompromised patients. Cl Microbiology Rev. 2007;20:695–704.
41. Odds FC. Candida and Candidosis. 2nd ed. London: Bailliere Tindall; 1988. p. 75.
42. Padhye AA, Smith G, Mc laughten D, et al. Comparative evaluation of a chemiluminescent DNA probe and an exoantigen test for rapid identification of H. Capsulatum. J Clin Microbiol. 1992;30:3108–11.
43. Pappagianis D. Epidemiology of coccidioidomycosis. Curr Top Med Mycol. 1988;2:199–238.
44. Parfrey NA. Improved diagnosis and prognosis of mucormycosis. A clinicopathologic study of 33 cases. Medicine. 1986;65:113–23.
45. Parker JC. The potentially lethal problem of cardiac candidiasis. Am J Clin Pathol. 1980;73:356–61.
46. Powderly WG, Cloud GA, Dismukes WE, et al. Measurement of cryptococcal antigen in serum and cerebrospinal fluid: value in the management of AIDS associated cryptococcal meningitis. Clin Infect Dis. 1994;18:789–92.
47. Stranger SL, Stringer JR, Blasé MA, Walzer PD, Cushion MT, et al. Pneumocystis carinii: sequence from ribosomal RNA implies a close relationship with fungi. Exp Parasitol. 1989;68:450–61.
48. Walsh TJ, Larone DH, Schell WA, Mitchell TG. Histoplasma, Blastomyces, Coccidioides and other dimorphic fungi causing systemic mycoses. In: Murray RP, Editor. Manual of clinical microbiology. 8th ed. Washington, DC: ASM Press; 2003.
49. Watts JC, Chandler FW. Aspergillosis. In: Connor DH, Cha FW, editors. Pathology of infectious diseases, vol. II. Stamford: Appleton & Lange; 1939.
50. Wheat LJ, Connolly-Springfield PA, Baker RL, et al. Disseminated histoplasmosis in the acquired immune deficiency syndrome: clinical findings, diagnosis and treatment and review of the literature. Medicine (Baltimore). 1990;69:361–74.
51. Yu VL, Moder RR, Poorsattar A. Significance of isolation of aspergillus from the respiratory tract in diagnosis of invasive pulmonary aspergillosis: result from a three-year prospective study. Am J Med. 1986;81:249–54.
52. Zaman MK, Wooter OJ, Suprahmanya B, et al. Rapid non invasive diagnosis of pneumocystis carinii from induced liquefied sputum. Am Intern Med. 1988;109:7–10.

5 Opportunistic Parasitic Infections

Immunocompromised patients present with altered pattern, progression, and clinical manifestations of parasitic infections. Patients with impaired cell-mediated immunity are susceptible to infection with *Toxoplasma gondii*, *Cryptosporidium*, *Leishmania*, *Strongyloides*, and *Microspora*. Defects in humoral immunity make the patient susceptible to infection by parasites like *Giardia lamblia* and *Cryptosporidium*. The immunocompromised patients are at risk of developing the following parasitic infections.

***Giardia lamblia*:** *G. lamblia* is a flagellated intestinal protozoon. Immunocompromised individuals are more susceptible to the development of chronic giardiasis. The organism is transmitted via fecal-oral route. Clinical manifestations are variable. Both cyst and trophozoite forms may be demonstrated in stool samples. Trophozoites of *Giardia* may be seen as pear-shaped, sickle, or crescent-shaped structures adhering to crypts of mucosal epithelium of the duodenum and proximal jejunum.

Table 5.1 Common opportunistic parasitic infections

Intestinal protozoa	Tissue protozoa	Hemoflagellates	Intestinal nematodes
Giardia lamblia	*Toxoplasma gondii*	*Leishmania*	*Strongyloides stercoralis*
Entamoeba			
Cryptosporidium parvum			
Cyclospora			
Isospora belli			
Sarcocystis			
Microsporidia			

From: Gupta RK. *Pathology of Opportunistic Infections in Tropics*. Jaypee; 2007

R.K. Gupta, P. Gupta (eds.), *Pathology of Opportunistic Infections*,
DOI 10.1007/978-981-10-1669-1_5

Giardiasis Duodenum in a Patient of Short Bowel Syndrome

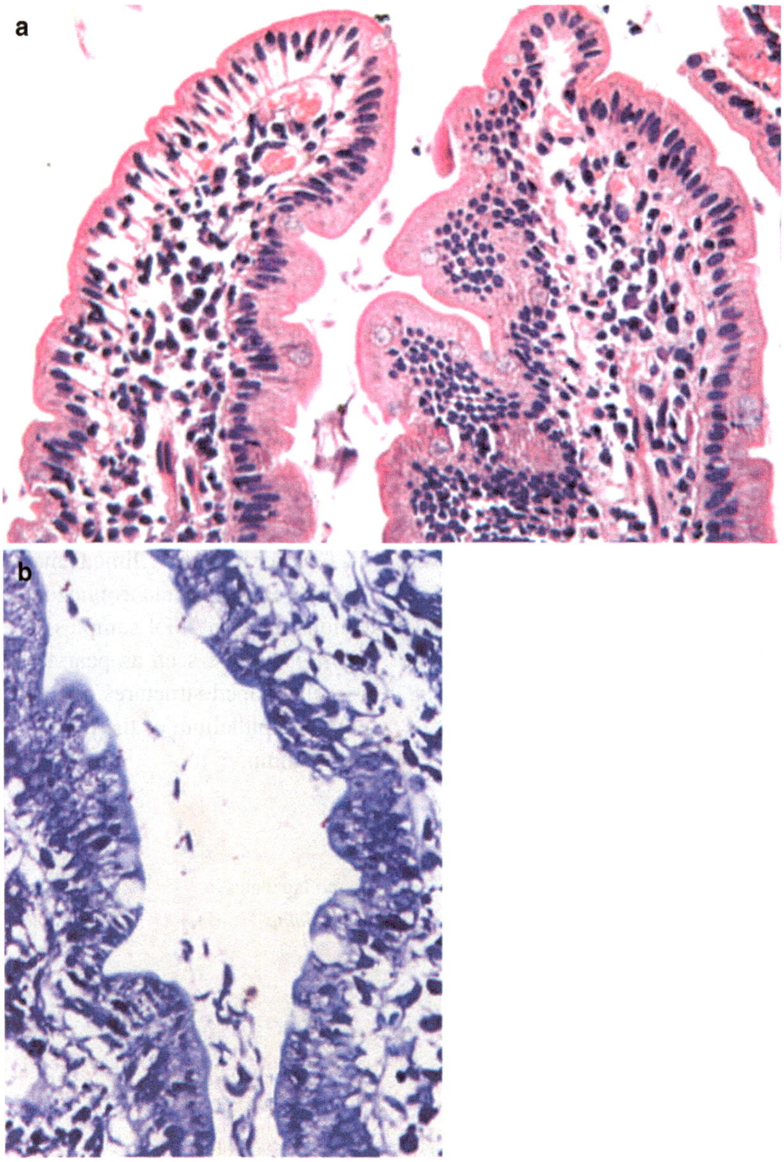

Fig. 5.1 (**a**, **b**) A 31-year-old male patient who underwent surgery for acute abdomen later presented with large volume watery diarrhea, extreme emaciation, and weight loss. On investigations he was found to have short bowel syndrome with the absence of a large length of the ileum. Duodenal biopsy revealed *Giardia* in the duodenal crypts suggesting giardiasis of the duodenum (**a** HE ×400 and **b** Giemsa ×400) (From: R K Gupta. *Pathology of Opportunistic Infections in Tropics*. Jaypee; 2007)

Entamoeba: *Entamoeba histolytica* is an intestinal protozoan parasite. Invasive amoebiasis is common in immunocompromised host. Primary amoebic encephalitis is caused by free-living amoeba, e.g., Naegleria, *Acanthamoeba*, and rarely *Balamuthia mandrillaris*. These amoebae are specifically neurotropic.

Acanthamoeba Brain

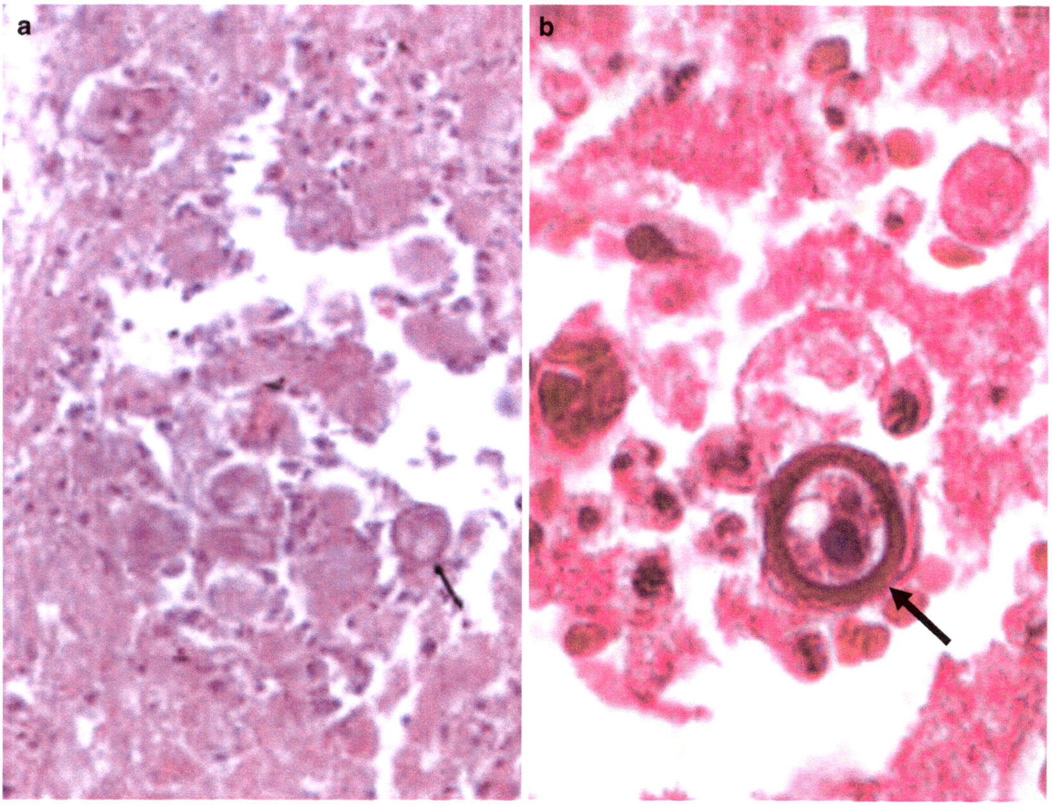

Fig. 5.2 (**a**, **b**) A 36-year-old agricultural worker was brought to the hospital with the history of fever, headache, vomiting, and cough with expectoration for 10 days. He had acidotic breathing and was drowsy. Clinical examination revealed right hemiparesis. Fundoscopy revealed bilateral papilledema. CSF examination revealed raised proteins and lymphocytic pleocytosis with occasional histiocytes. He had three episodes of seizures on the sixth day of admission followed by cardiopulmonary arrest to which he succumbed. At postmortem the gross examination of the brain showed areas of hemorrhagic infarct in the frontal lobe. Histological examination revealed necrotic tissue with the presence of a few large trophozoites and cyst of *Acanthomoeba* (**a** HE ×400 and **b** PAS ×1000) (Contributors: Dr. Anita Mahadevan and Prof. S K Shankar, Human Brain Bank, Department of Neuropathology, NIMHANS, Bangalore) (From: R K Gupta. *Pathology of opportunistic infections in tropics*. Jaypee; 2007)

***Balantidium coli*:** It is a ciliated protozoan causing zoonotic infection. Pig is an important natural reservoir. The infection is transmitted to man through food and water contaminated by fecal matter of pig. Infection in man could both be intestinal and extraintestinal. It is the largest protozoa; the trophozoites have granular cytoplasm with two nuclei, one bean-shaped macronucleus, and a small micronucleus.

Balantidium coli in a Cavitary Lung Lesion in an Immunocompromised Patient

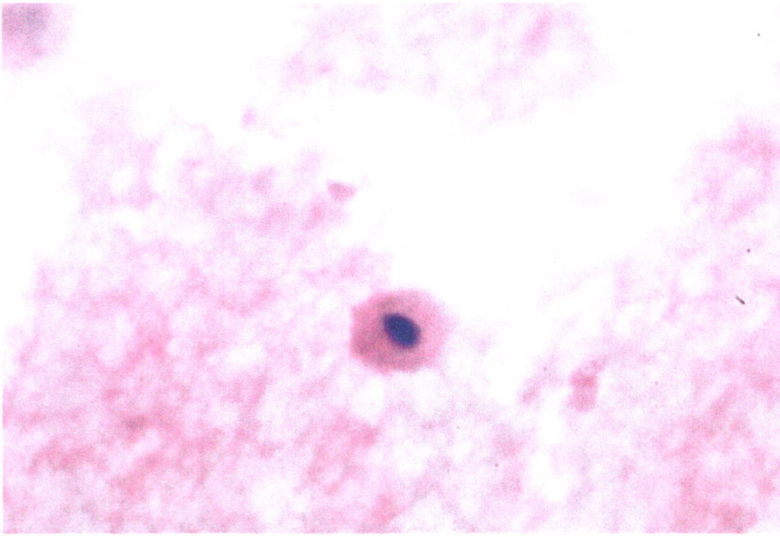

Fig. 5.3 A 23-year-old male Indian national studying medicine in Russia presented with swelling all over the body for 4 months along with nausea, vomiting, and hiccups for 2 days. Serum creatinine was 8.9 mg/dl and blood urea 178 mg/dl; urine examination revealed active sediment. He was on steroids for 10 months and was HIV negative. X-ray chest revealed a cavitary lesion in the basal segment of the left lung. Guided FNAC of the lung revealed large round- to oval-ciliated structures with an eccentrically placed reniform nucleus, the background showed necrotic debris (HE ×400). Wet preparation showed that these organisms were actively motile with cilia suggestive of trophozoites of *Balantidium coli*. Stains for AFB and fungus were negative. Renal biopsy showed amyloidosis (Contributors: Dr. S. Radha and Dr. Tameem Afroz, Department of Pathology, Aware Global Hospital, Hyderabad, India) (From: R K Gupta. *Pathology of Opportunistic Infections in Tropics*. Jaypee; 2007)

Cryptosporidium: *Cryptosporium parvum* is an intestinal protozoan. It is one of the common opportunistic infections in patients of AIDS. Immunocompromised patients present with severe prolonged diarrhea with fatal outcome. The infection is transmitted from animals or person to person contact through fecal-oral route. The *Cryptosporidium* infects the mucosa of the gastrointestinal tract with the jejunum being the most heavily infected site. The sporozoites attach to the apical membrane of enterocytes. Duodenal/jejunal mucosal biopsy shows small rounded organisms (1–3 μm).

Cryptosporidiosis Duodenum in a HIV-Positive Patient

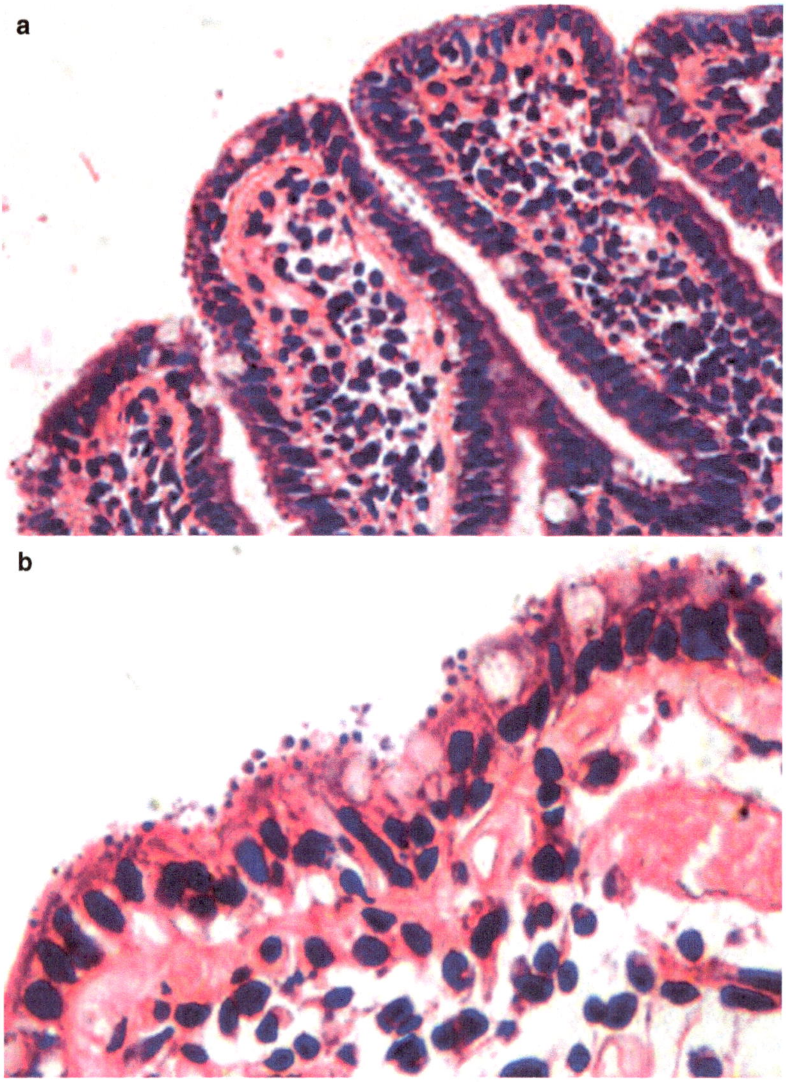

Fig. 5.4 (**a**, **b**) A 56-year-old female patient with history of blood transfusion from a professional donor for an ovarian surgery 8 years back presented with increased frequency of stools, large volume watery diarrhea, occasional vomiting, loss of weight, and fever. Upper GI endoscopy revealed nodularity in the upper esophagus and stomach. Duodenal biopsy showed partial villous atrophy with the presence of small rounded organisms of *Cryptosporidium* closely apposed to the surface epithelium (**a** HE ×400, **b** HE ×1000). Gastric biopsy also showed *Cytomegalovirus* infection. The patient was HIV positive with absolute CD4 count of 138 cells/μl (From: R K Gupta. *Pathology of Opportunistic Infections in Tropics*. Jaypee; 2007)

Cryptosporidiosis Colon in a Renal Allograft Recipient

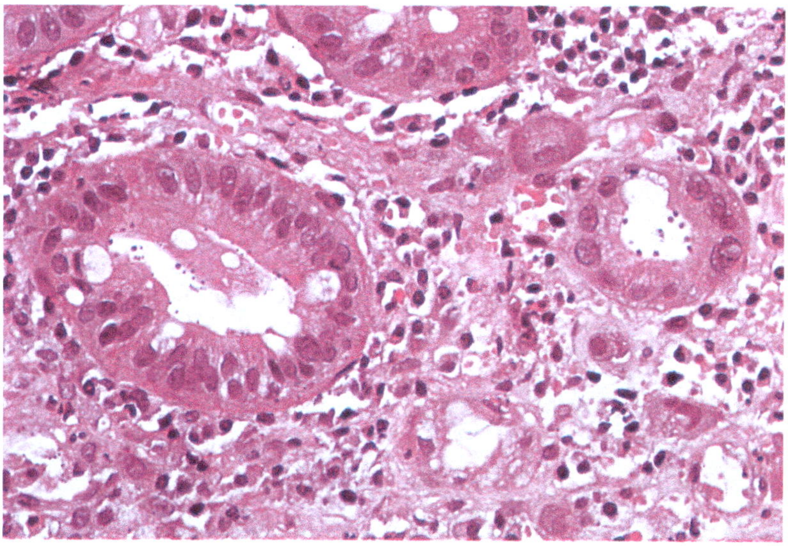

Fig. 5.5 A 42-year-old male receiving live-related renal allograft, 2 years posttransplant, presented with loose stools and vomiting for 10 days. Routine laboratory workup and USG abdomen were WNL. Graft was otherwise well functioning with serum creatinine level of 1.12 mg/dl. Colonoscopic examination revealed erythematous spots throughout the colon. Endoscopic biopsy revealed the presence of *Cryptosporidium* adhering to crypt epithelium (HE ×400)

Isospora belli: *Isospora* are coccidian parasites, which do not have an intermediate host. Man acts as a definitive host where both sexual and asexual cycles take place. Isosporiasis is endemic worldwide. The infection is acquired by the intake of contaminated food and water containing mature oocysts.

It is an important opportunistic infection being increasingly recognized in patients with HIV/AIDS, more commonly in homosexuals. The patients present with chronic diarrhea and debilitation. In severe cases the disease could be fatal. Peripheral blood eosinophilia is usually present. Duodenal biopsy may show intracellular stages of the organism. Fresh stool samples and duodenal aspirates may show oocysts. Modified acid-fast stain is useful in identification of the oocysts.

Isosporiasis in a Child on Prolonged Steroid Therapy

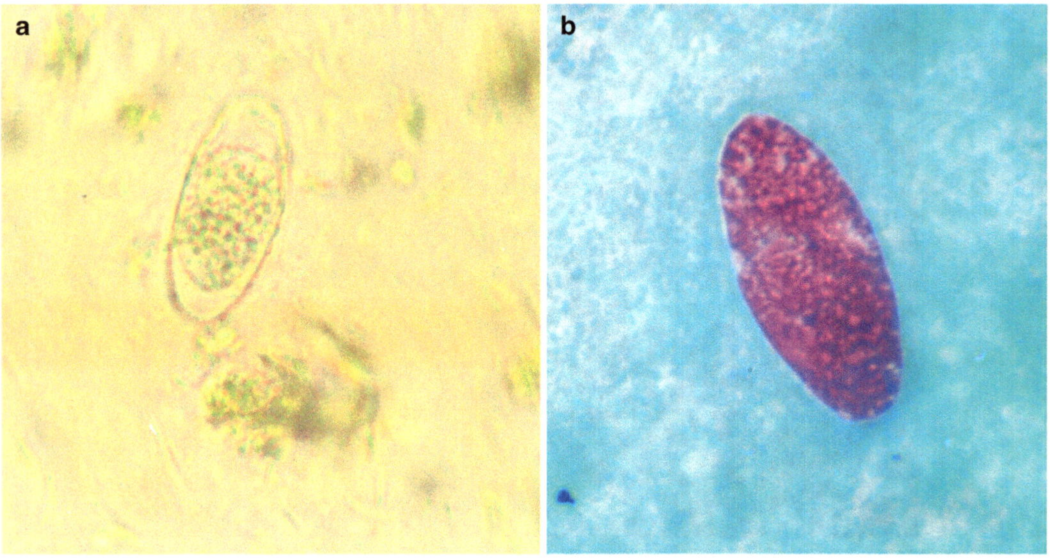

Fig. 5.6 (**a**, **b**) A 2-year-old male child was receiving low-dose steroid therapy for Budd-Chiari syndrome for the past 8 months. He was admitted to the hospital with complaint of severe diarrhea for 1 week. The stool was watery with a frequency of 15–20 stools a day. He also had low-grade fever, intermittent productive cough, and oral candidiasis. Routine hematological and biochemical lab profiles were within normal limits. HIV ELISA performed twice was negative. Serum C3 was 11.68 mg/dl and serum IgA was 89 mg/dl. Anti-Sm antibodies were present. CD4 count was 330 cells/µl. Stool examination showed oocysts of *Isospora* (20–25/hpf) (**a** wet iodine mount ×400 and **b** modified Ziehl-Neelsen stain ×1000). Initially the patient responded to co-trimoxazole therapy; however he subsequently developed recurrence of isosporiasis with protein allergy malnutrition (grade III). He also developed allergy to co-trimoxazole and died after a period of 5 months (Contributor: Dr Vipul Kumar Srivastava, Consultant Microbiologist, Sahara Hospital, Lucknow, India)

***Toxoplasma gondii*:** It is an obligate intracellular tissue protozoan. Symptomatic infection is seen only in immunocompromised states or in infants with congenital infection. Important predisposing conditions are AIDS, organ transplant recipients, and hematopoietic malignancies. Individuals with CD4 count less than 100/ul are at increased risk.

Cats are definitive host. Man is infected by ingestion of cysts. Transplacental transmission may also occur. Although systemic toxoplasmosis may affect any organ, Toxoplasma encephalitis is the most common. Tissue biopsy may be performed to demonstrate the organisms. Intracellular parasite in the form of both cysts and trophozoites is found. Direct immunofluorescence, immunohistochemistry, and PCR can also be performed on paraffin-embedded tissue.

Toxoplasma Colon (Disseminated Toxoplasmosis) in a Renal Allograft Recipient

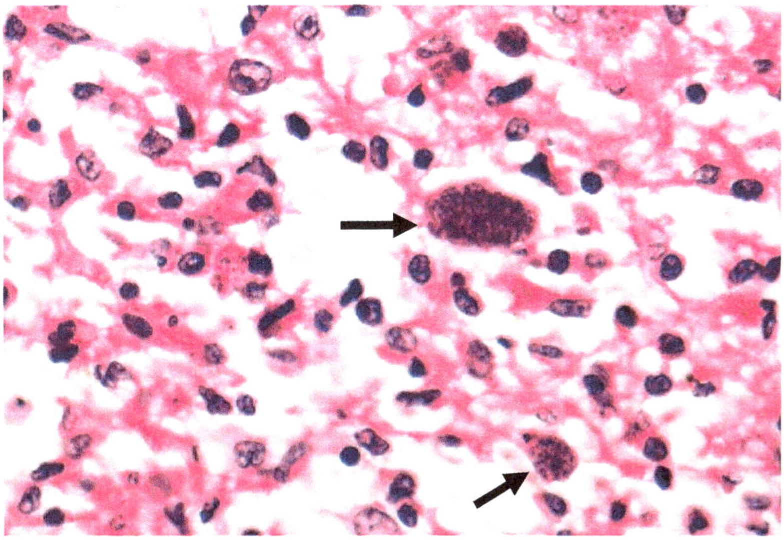

Fig. 5.7 A 35-year-old male patient who received a live-related renal allograft 3 months back presented with acute colitis, CSOM (otomycosis), and altered sensorium. Colonic biopsy revealed cysts of *Toxoplasma* (HE ×400) (Contributor – Prof. Kusum Joshi, Postgraduate Institute of Medical Education and Research, Chandigarh, India) (From: R K Gupta. *Pathology of Opportunistic Infections in Tropics*. Jaypee; 2007)

Toxoplasma Brain in a HIV-Positive Patient

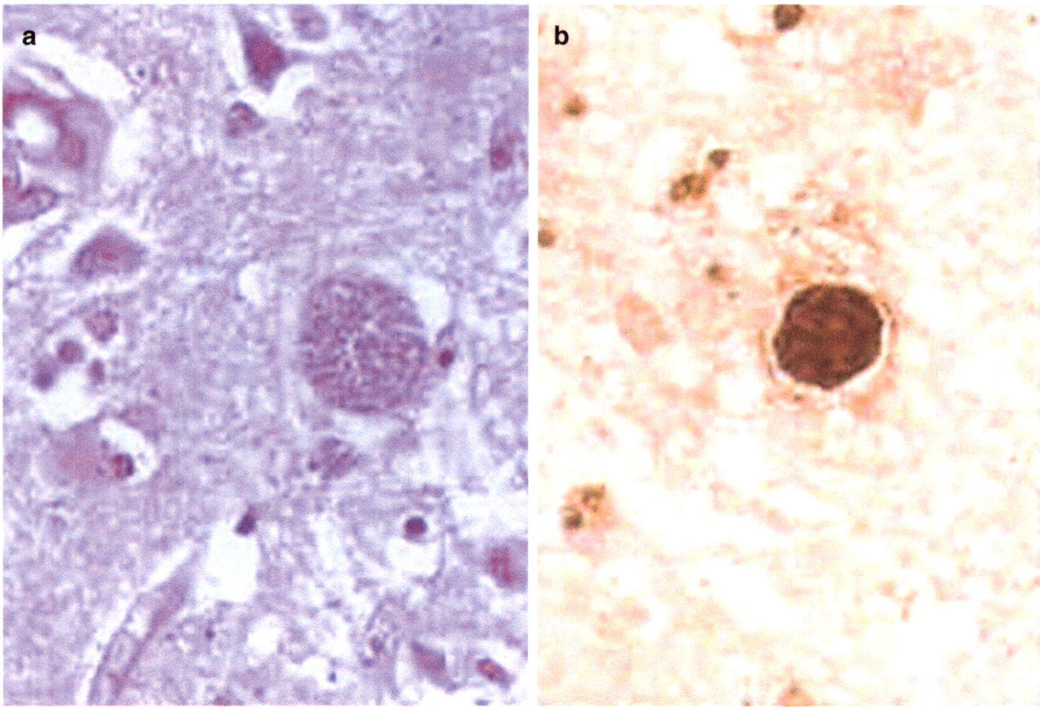

Fig. 5.8 (**a**, **b**) A 32-year-old female patient complaining of headache, vomiting, generalized fatigue, and intermittent fever, mainly at night for 1 month presented with ataxia and altered sensorium for 10 days. She has undergone hysterectomy 4 years back and received two units of blood transfusion. Neurological examination revealed features of meningitis and lower cranial nerve involvement. Cranial CT revealed bilateral multiple hypodense lesions in parieto-occipital region, right corona radiata, and left temporal lobe. CSF examination revealed proteins, 70 mg%; sugar, 82 mg%; and lymphocytic pleocytosis. India ink preparation was negative for cryptococci; CSF was also negative for antimycobacterial antibody. *Toxoplasma gondii* antibodies were present both in serum and CSF. Clinical diagnosis of cerebral toxoplasmosis was made, and appropriate antibiotic therapy was initiated. Patient deteriorated rapidly and succumbed. Postmortem serum sample was detected to be reactive for HIV 1 (by three test procedures). Postmortem brain histology showed cysts and tachyzoites of *Toxoplasma* (**a** HE ×400, **b** Mason Fontana ×400) (Contributors – Dr. Anita Mahadevan and Prof. S K Shankar, Human Brain Bank, Dept. of Neuropathology, NIMHANS, Bangalore, India) (From: R K Gupta. *Pathology of Opportunistic Infections in Tropics*. Jaypee; 2007)

***Leishmania* (Causative Agent of Leishmaniasis):** *Leishmania* is an obligate intracellular protozoon. Visceral leishmaniasis has emerged as an opportunistic infection in patients of AIDS, transplant recipients, and other immunocompromised states associated with suppressed cell-mediated immunity. It is a vector-borne zoonotic infection transmitted by the bite of female phlebotomine sand fly. The disease is also transmitted transplacentally and parenterally. In patients with HIV infection, besides hepatosplenomegaly, other organs like GIT, lung, pleura, and oral mucosa may also be involved. Certain atypical presentations are observed in patients of AIDS. They may remain asymptomatic, hepatosplenomegaly may not be seen, and the patients may present with aplastic anemia due to bone marrow involvement. Diagnosis of leishmaniasis is established by the demonstration of intracellular amastigotes in the macrophages. PCR and other molecular techniques are being increasingly used for identification of parasite.

Leishmania Bone Marrow in a Renal Allograft Recipient

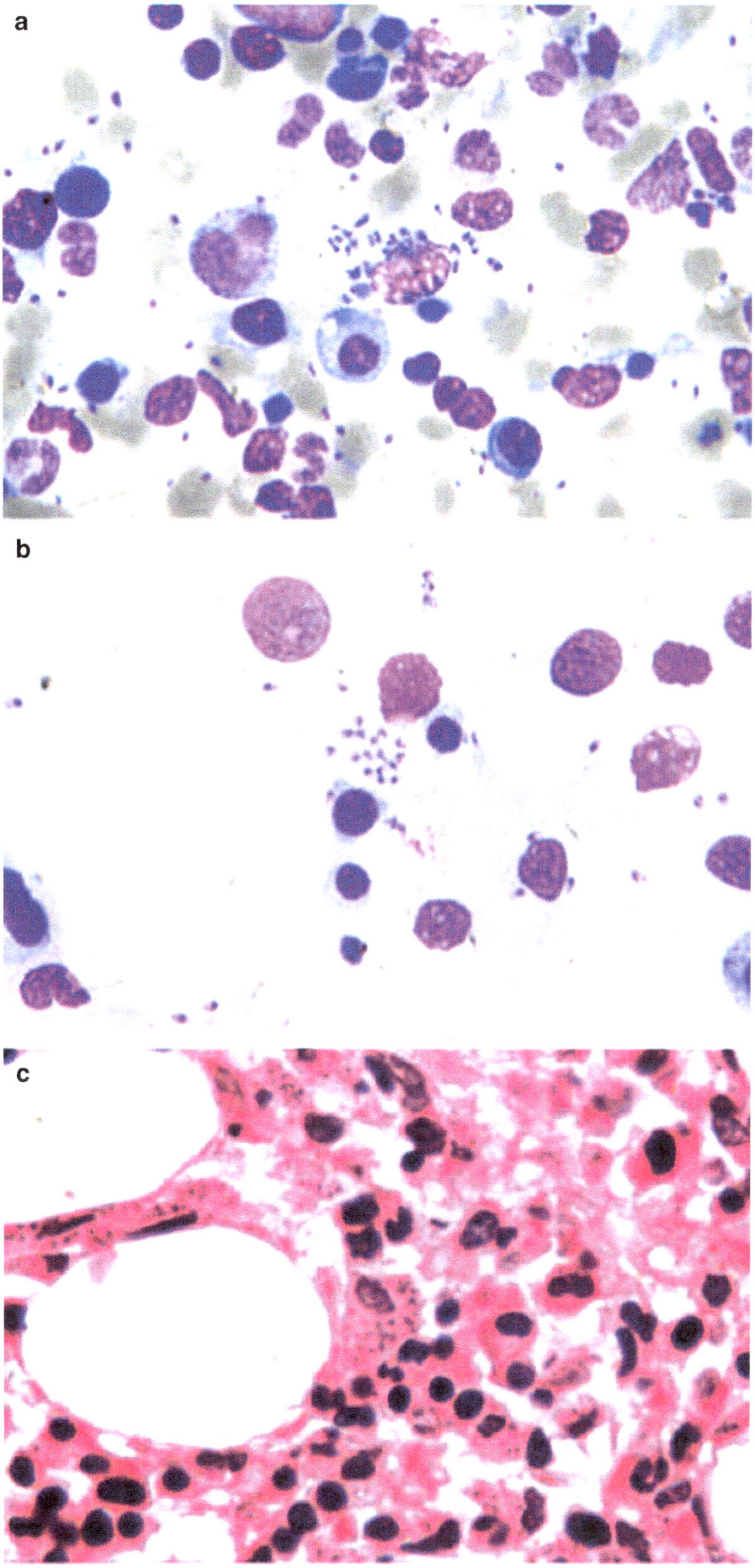

Fig. 5.9 (**a**, **b**) A 35-year-old male renal allograft recipient, 7 years posttransplant, presented with PUO. Investigations revealed anemia and leukopenia and deteriorating renal functions. Bone marrow aspirate revealed plasmacytosis and presence of LD bodies in RE cells; extracellular LD bodies were also seen (**a**, **b** Leishman stain ×1000). Bone marrow biopsy also showed similar findings (**c** HE ×1000) (From: R K Gupta. *Pathology of Opportunistic Infections in Tropics*. Jaypee; 2007)

***Strongyloides stercoralis* (Commonly Known as Thread Worm, Causative Agent of Strongyloidosis):** *Strongyloides stercoralis* is an intestinal nematode with a dual life cycle and can perpetuate both in the soil and the host. Immunocompromised states such as transplant recipients, prolonged corticosteroid therapy, and patients of malignancy have increased risk of autoinfection, thereby causing hyperinfection. Uncontrolled hyperinfection may lead to dissemination of organisms to extraintestinal sites such as the lungs, CNS, liver, kidney, and peritoneum. AIDS is not associated with increased predisposition to strongyloidosis. In immunocompromised patients the duodenal biopsy shows large number of parasites buried in the crypts. Rhabditiform larvae are found in the stools.

Strongyloides stercoralis (Duodenal Biopsy) in a Renal Allograft Recipient

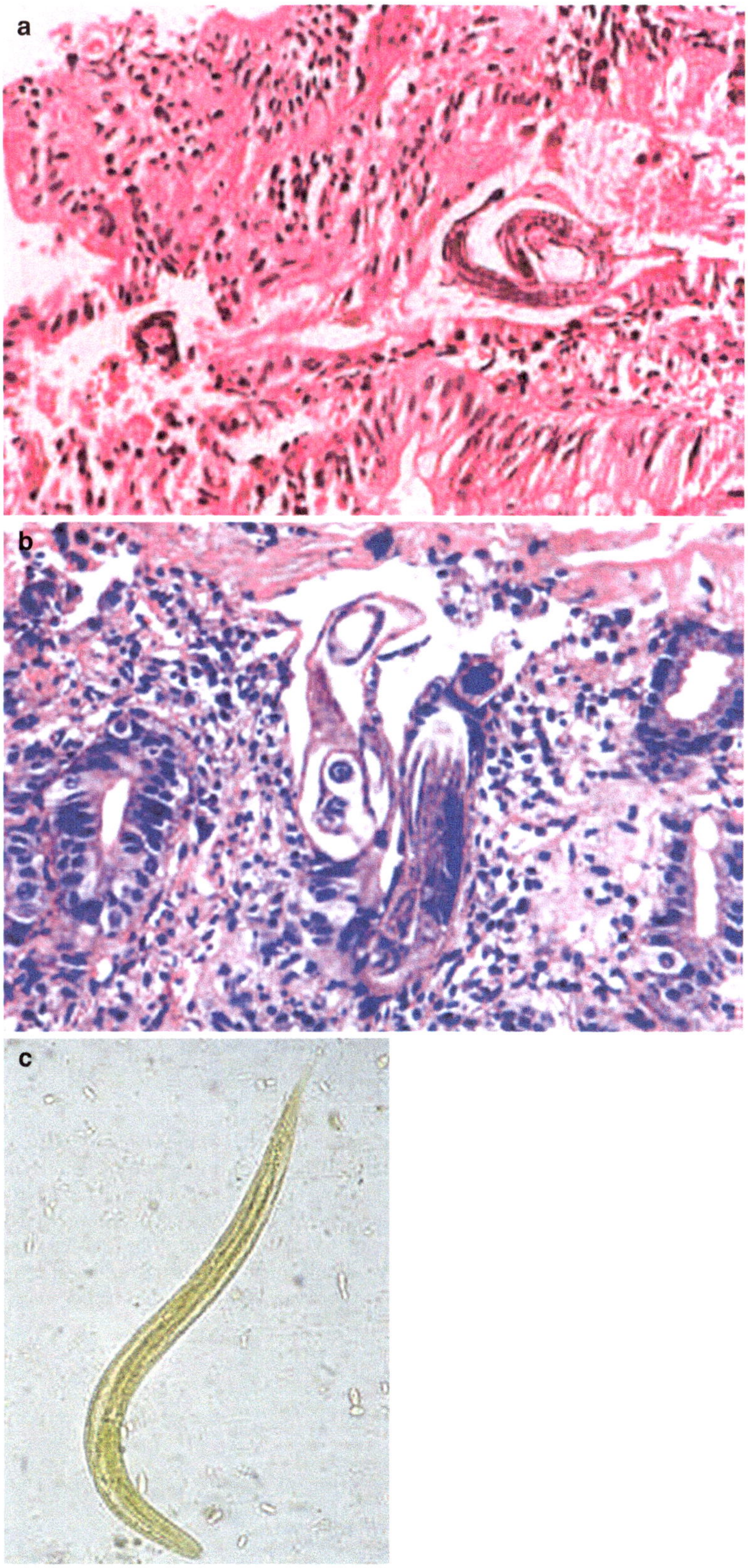

Fig. 5.10 (**a**–**c**) A 33-year-old male renal allograft recipient presented 10 months posttransplant with malabsorption syndrome. Upper GI endoscopy showed nodularity in duodenal mucosa. Histological examination of duodenal biopsy showed subtotal villous atrophy and multiple larvae of *Strongyloides* in the mucosa (**a**, **b** HE ×400). The stool examination also showed rhabditiform larvae of *Strongyloides* (**c** wet iodine mount ×400) (From: R K Gupta. *Pathology of Opportunistic Infections in Tropics*. Jaypee; 2007)

Strongyloides stercoralis (Duodenal Biopsy) in a Patient of Chronic Liver Disease

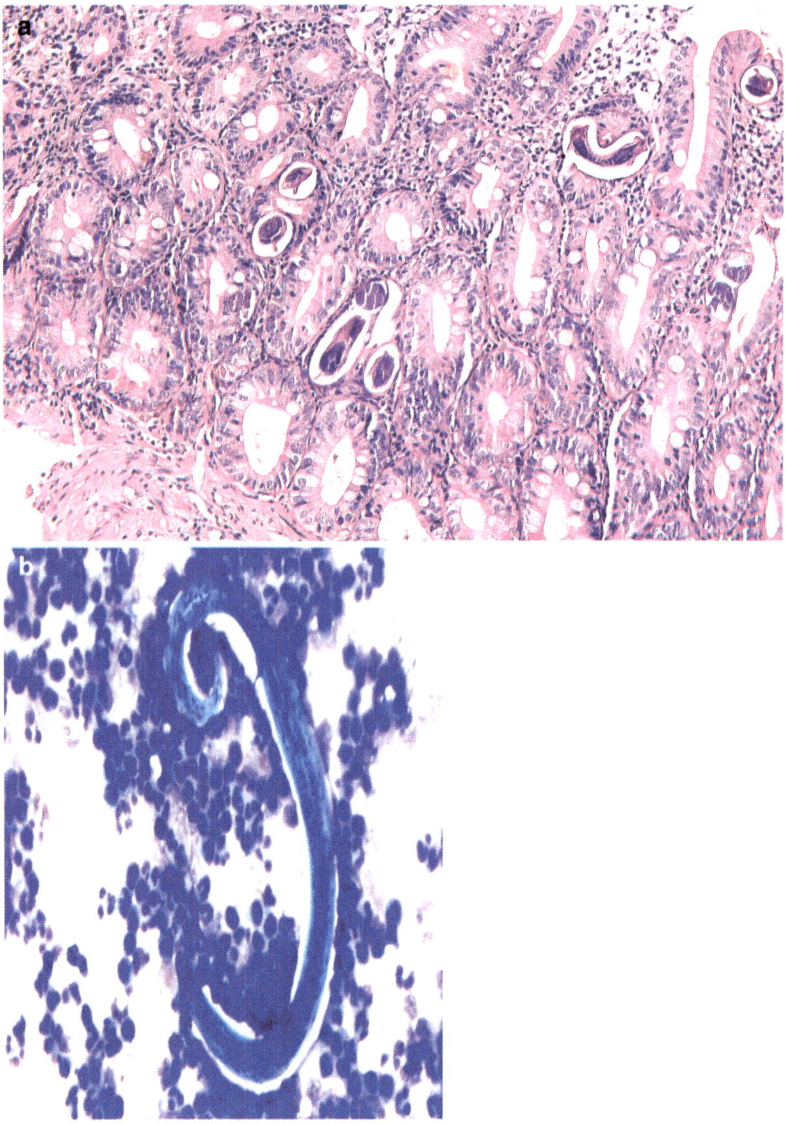

Fig. 5.11 (**a**, **b**) A 66-year-old male admitted as a case of chronic liver disease with ascites and grade III hepatic encephalopathy underwent upper GI endoscopy, which revealed duodenal (d2) nodularity. The duodenal biopsy (**a** HE ×400) revealed the presence of larvae of *Strongyloides*. Cytological examination of ascitic fluid cytospin smears also showed the presence of larvae of *Strongyloides* (**b** MGG ×400). The presence of the parasite in the ascitic fluid could be explained by autoinfection. Autoinfection results from conversion of rhabditiform larvae into filariform larvae in the intestine and then penetration of the intestinal wall by infective larvae which may reach the peritoneal cavity (From: R K Gupta. *Pathology of Opportunistic Infections in Tropics*. Jaypee; 2007)

Further Reading

1. Alvar J, Cavavate C, Gutierrez-Solar BA. Leishmania and human immunodeficiency virus coinfection: the first 10 years. Clin Microbiol Rev. 1997;10:298–319.
2. Beaver PC, Jung RC, Cupp EW. Clinical parasitology. 9th ed. Philadelphia: Lea & Febeger; 1984.
3. Butt CG. Primary amebic meningoencephalitis. N Engl J Med. 1966;274:1473–6.
4. Donovan C. On the possibility of the occurrence of trypanosomiasis in India. Br Med J. 1903;2:79.
5. Gellin BG, Soave R. Coccidian infections in AIDS: toxoplasmosis, cryptosporidiosis and isosporiasis. Med Clin North Am. 1992;76:205–34.
6. Gupta RK. Opportunistic infections in renal allograft recipients. Transplant Proc. 2007;39:731–3.
7. Gupta RK. Opportunistic parasitic infections. In: Pathology of opportunistic infections in tropics. New Delhi: Jaypee; 2007. p. 70.
8. Hoge CW, Shlim DR, Rajah R, Triplett J, Shear M, Rabold JH, et al. Epidemiology of diarrhoeal illness associated with coccidian like organism among travelers and foreign residents in Nepal. N Engl J Med. 1993;341:1175–9.
9. Israelski DM, Chmiel JS, Poggensee L, Phair JP, Remington JS. Prevalence of Toxoplasma infection in a cohort of homosexual men at risk of AIDS and toxoplasmic encephalitis. J Acq Immuno Defic Syndr. 1993;6:414–8.
10. Fowler M, Carter RF. Acute pyogenic meningitis probably due to Acanthamoeba species: a preliminary report. Br Med J. 1965;5464:740–2.
11. Kahn DJ, Garfinkle JM, Klonoff DC, Pembrook LJ, Marrow DJ. Cryptosporidial and cytomegaloviral hepatitis and cholecystitis. Arch Pathol Lab Med. 1987;111:879–81.
12. Leishman WB. On the possibility of the occurrence of trypanosomiasis in India. Br Med J. 1903;2:1252–4.
13. Lucas SB. Missing infection in AIDS. Trans R Soc Trop Med Hyg. 1990;84:34–88.
14. Medrano FJ, Jimenez Mejas E, Calderon E, Regordan C, Leal M. Correspondence. An easy and quick method for the diagnosis of visceral leishmaniasis in HIV-1 infected individuals. AIDS. 1993;7(10):1399.
15. Moore JA, Frenkel JK. Respiratory and enteric cryptosporidiosis in humans. Arch Pathol Lab Med. 1991;115:1160–2.
16. Moulin B, Olier J, Bouchouareb D, Pwrgus R, Olner M. Leishmaniasis: a rare cause of unexplained fever in a renal graft recipient. Nephron. 1992;60:360–2.
17. Murray JF, Garay SM, Hopewell PC, et al. NHLB Workshop summary: pulmonary complications of the acquired immunodeficiency syndrome. An update. Am Rev Resp Dis. 1987;135:504–9.
18. Nhieu JIV, Nin F, Fleury Feith J, et al. Identification of intracellular stages of cyclospora species by light microscopy of thick sections using Hematoxylin. Hum Pathol. 1996;27:1107–9.
19. Pieniazek NJ, Slemenda SB, De Silva AJ, Alfano EM, Arrowood MJ. PCR confirmation of Infection with Cyclospora cayetanensis. Emerging Infect Dis. 1996; 2:357–8.
20. Restrepo C, Macher AM, Radany EH. Disseminated extraintestinal isosporiasis in a patient with acquired immune deficiency syndrome. Am J Clin Pathol. 1987;87:536–42.
21. Ross R. (1) Note on the bodies recently described by Leishman and Donovan and (2) further notes on Leishman's bodies. Br Med J. 1903;2:1261–401.
22. Wurtz R. Cyclospora: a newly identified pathogen of humans. Clin Infect Dis. 1994;18:620–3.

6 Multiple Opportunistic Infections

Fungal infections constitute the largest group of opportunistic infections, followed by others such as bacterial, viral, and parasitic. Majority of immunocompromised patients experience opportunistic infection by a single pathogen; however, at times some of these patients may have multiple infections with more than one pathogen(s) (Table 6.1).

Table 6.1 Multiple opportunistic infections in immunocompromised patients

Case	First pathogen	Second pathogen	Site of first pathogen	Site of second pathogen	Cause of immunosuppression
1	*M. tuberculosis*	*Aspergillus* sp.	Subcutaneous tissue	Subcutaneous tissue	Steroids
2	H. zoster	*Candida* sp.	Esophagus	Esophagus	Renal transplant
3	CMV	*Aspergillus* sp.	Renal allograft	Renal allograft	Renal transplant
4	CMV	*Aspergillus* sp.	Stomach	Subcutaneous tissue (greater toe)	Renal transplant
5	CMV	PTLD	Stomach	Stomach	Renal transplant
6	CMV	*Cryptosporidium*	Esophagus	Duodenum	HIV
7	CMV	*Cryptosporidium*	Stomach	Stomach	HIV
8	Condyloma acuminatum	*H. capsulatum*	Vulvovaginal area	Cervical lymph nodes	SUHSIS
9	*Aspergillus*	*Candida*	Nasal polyp	Nasal polyp	Recurrent infection
10	*Zygomycetes*	*Candida* sp.	Paranasal sinus	Subcutaneous tissue	ALL
11	*Zygomycetes*	*Candida* sp.	Oral mucosa	Oral mucosa	ALL
12	*Mucor*	*Candida* sp.	Soft palate	Soft palate	Debilitating illness
13	*Zygomycetes*	*Acanthamoeba*	Brain	Brain	Herpes infection
14	*Strongyloides*	*Candida* sp.	Duodenum	Esophagus	Steroids
15	*Strongyloides*	*Giardia*	Duodenum	Duodenum	Steroids
16	*Giardia*	*Candida* sp.	Duodenum	Stomach	Renal transplant

R.K. Gupta, P. Gupta (eds.), *Pathology of Opportunistic Infections*,
DOI 10.1007/978-981-10-1669-1_6

CMV Gastritis with Cryptosporidiosis Stomach in a HIV-Positive Patient

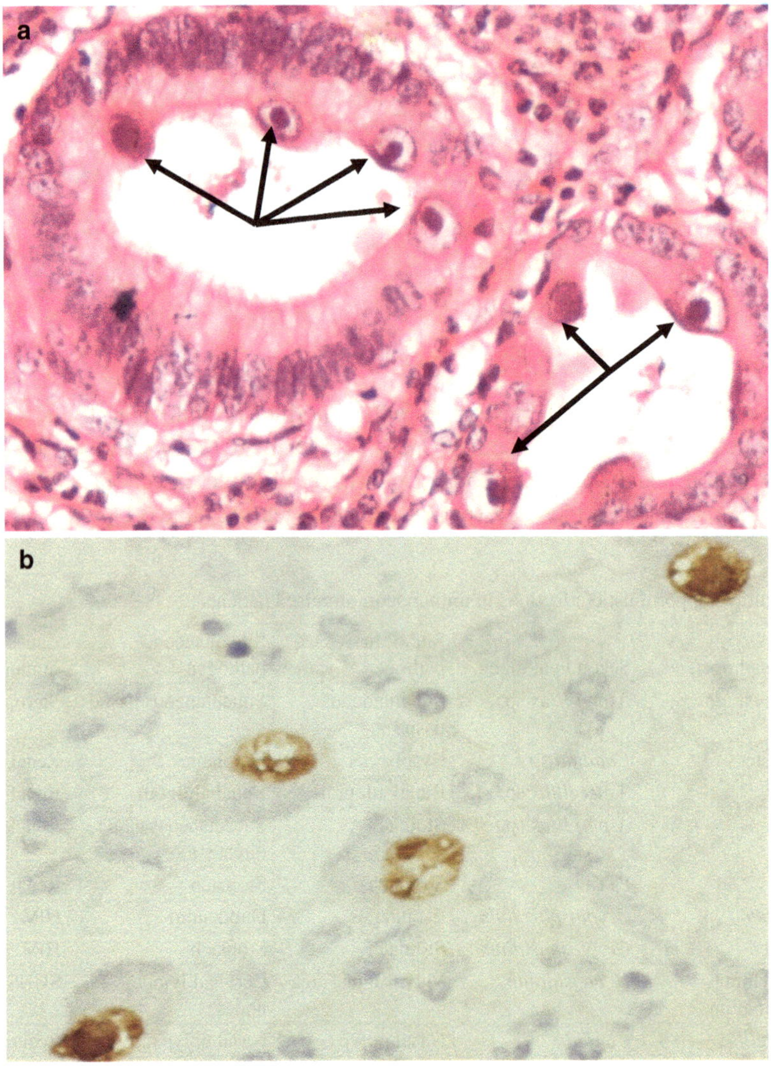

Fig. 6.1 (**a**–**c**) A 49-year-old male patient presented with 1-month history of epigastric discomfort, loose stools, painful perianal swelling, productive cough, marked loss of appetite, and loss of weight. Routine hematological and biochemical laboratory investigations were within normal limits. X-ray chest, USG abdomen, and CT scan were also not contributory. Upper GI endoscopy showed candidal esophagitis, distortion of gastric folds in the body, and the antrum with flat ulcerated lesions. Histopathological examination of endoscopic gastric biopsy showed marked architectural distortion and nuclear pleomorphism of gastric glands. On this endoscopic biopsy, histopathological diagnosis of adenocarcinoma stomach was offered. Gastrectomy was performed. The gastrectomy specimen showed a 5 × 3 × 1.5 cm growth, 3 cm distal to resected antral region. The overlying mucosa was flattened with focal areas of congestion and ulceration. Histological examination showed ulcerated gastric mucosa. The gastric glands adjacent to the ulcerated areas showed disorganization and stratification suggestive of psuedoadenomatous hyperplasia along with reactive atypia of lining epithelial cells of gastric mucosa. The gastric mucosa also showed CMV gastritis along with concomitant infestation by *Cryptosporidium* as another opportunistic infection. On subsequent investigations the patient was found to be HIV positive (**a** HE ×400, **b** IHC for CMV ×400 and **c** HE ×1000) (Contributor: Prof Harsh Mohan, Head of Department Pathology, Government Medical College, Chandigarh, India)

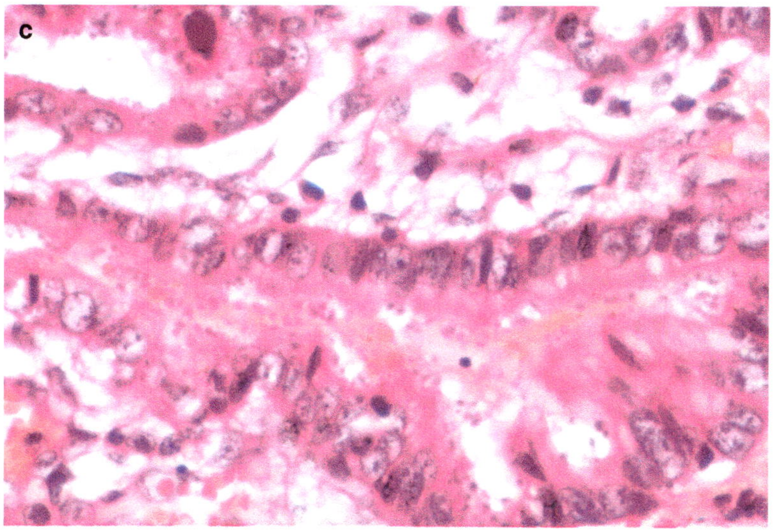

Fig. 6.1 (continued)

CMV Gastritis with Subcutaneous Aspergillosis in a Renal Allograft Recipient

Fig. 6.2 (**a–d**) A 25-year-old male patient receiving live-related renal allograft, 6 months posttransplant presented with vomiting for 2 days along with fever for 1 day and decreased in urine output. Serum creatinine was 2.7 mg/dl. Upper GI endoscopy revealed superficial multiple ulcerations in the fundal area, and gastric mucosa biopsy revealed CMV gastritis (**a**, **b** HE ×400). Subsequently he developed a swelling on the right foot. The FNAC revealed few acute angle branching septate hyphae with thin parallel walls, suggestive of *Aspergillus* (*arrows*) (**c** PAS ×400, **d** CSM ×400)

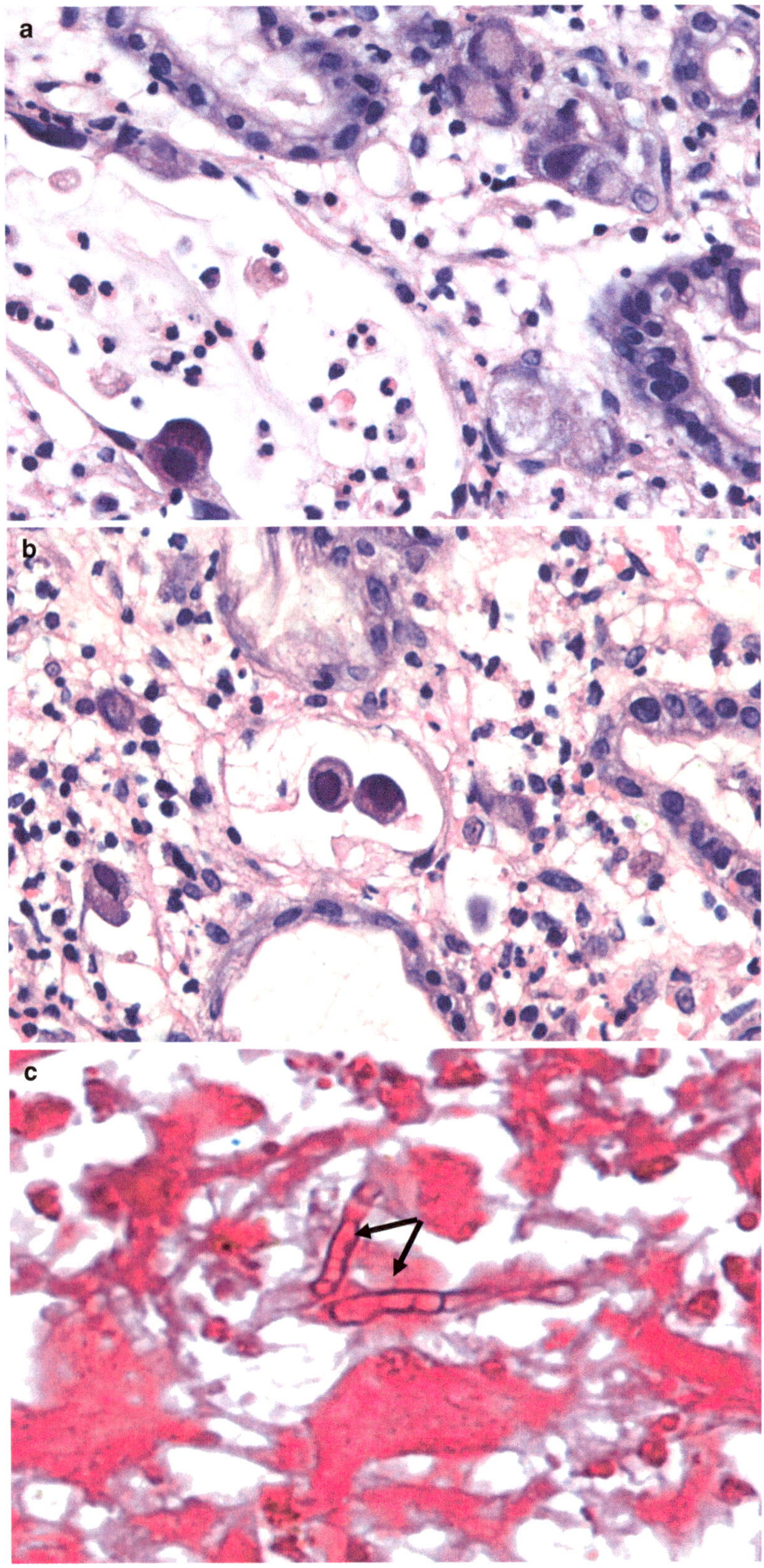

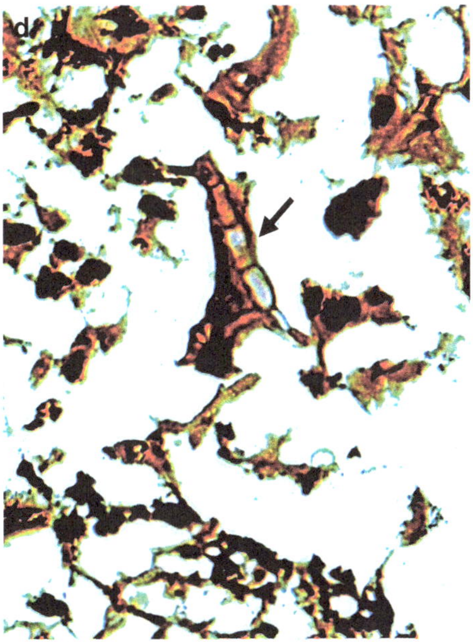

Fig. 6.2 (continued)

CMV with Aspergillosis Kidney in a Renal Allograft Recipient

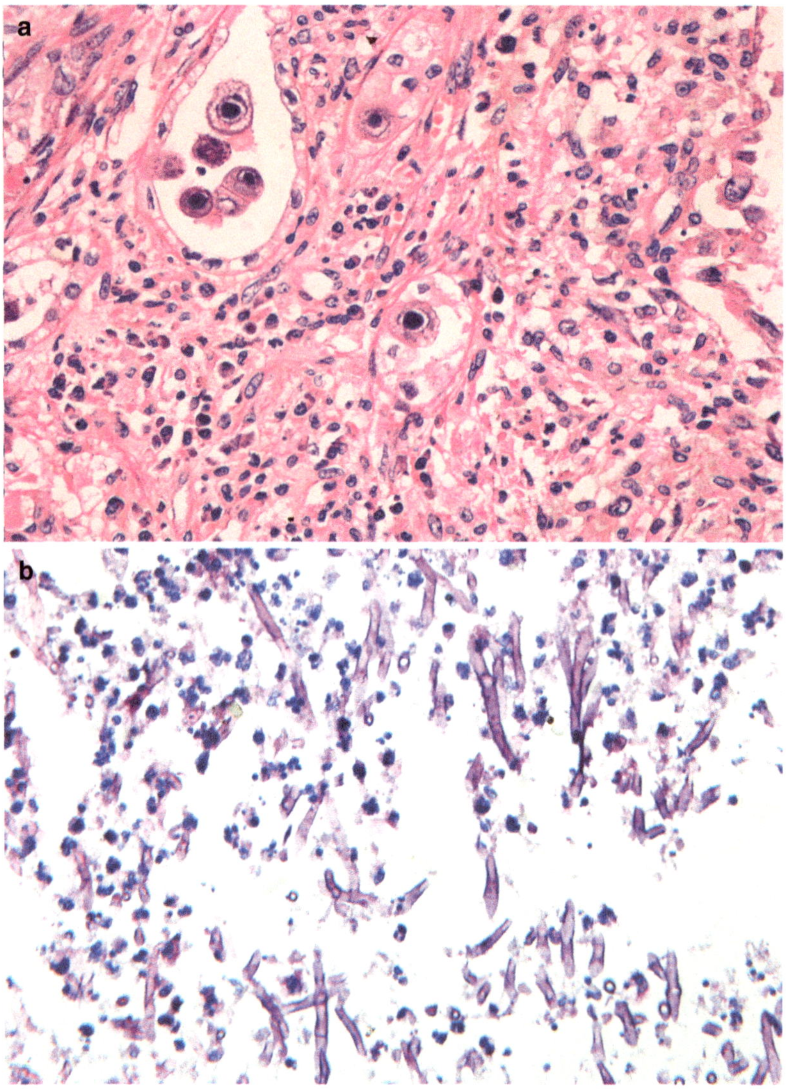

Fig. 6.3 (**a**, **b**) A 45-year-old female renal allograft recipient, presented with drop in urinary output, weakness, and anorexia on the seventh posttransplant day and was clinically diagnosed as acute rejection which responded to antirejection therapy. Three months later she again presented with rise in serum creatinine; USG of the renal allograft revealed fungal ball in the renal pelvis. In view of the infected graft, graft nephrectomy was performed. Histological evaluation showed severe tubulointerstitial nephritis with the presence of CMV kidney disease along with multiple microabscesses which revealed the presence of uniform septate acute angle branching fungal hyphae suggestive of *Aspergillus* (**a** HE ×400 and **b** PAS ×400)

Condyloma Acuminatum Along with Histoplasmosis Lymph Node in a Case of Severe Unexplained HIV Seronegative Immune Suppression (SUHSIS): Idiopathic CD4 Lymphocytopenia

a

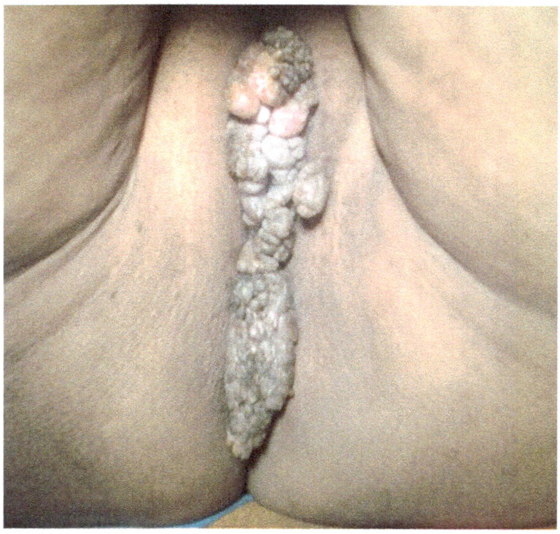

Fig. 6.4 (**a**–**l**) A 45-year-old female patient presented with bilateral cervical (including postauricular) and axillary lymphadenopathy for 2 months associated with intermittent low-grade pyrexia (99–100 °F). She had been suffering with oral mucosal ulcerations for the past 15 years, and she also had rashes with itching on both upper limbs for 5 years. She also had multiple warts in the vulval and perianal area for about 5 years. She had been receiving homeopathic treatment without significant improvement. Her social history was pertinent that her husband was in a job at a distant place and periodically visiting his family; however of late she had been living a separated life for about 6 years. Clinical examination revealed enlargement of bilateral cervical (more marked on the left side) and axillary lymph nodes, largest measuring 5 cm, they were soft to firm and non-matted; the left tonsil was also enlarged. Gynecological examination revealed multiple warts in vulvovaginal and perianal areas. X-ray chest was WNL; ultrasound abdomen did not reveal any organomegaly. Hematological workup showed hemoglobin of 11.7 g/dl, total WBC 6700/cu mm, differential WBC count showed relative lymphopenia with 18 % lymphocytes (absolute lymphocyte count: 1206/cu mm), and other hematology parameters were WNL. Bone marrow examination did not reveal any abnormality. The patient was nondiabetic, and the liver and renal function tests were not deranged. She was seronegative for HIV 1 and 2; however her CD 4 count was 345/cu mm. Serology for ANA, DsDNA, and ANCA was negative. Biopsy from the vulvovaginal warts was suggestive of condyloma acuminatum (**a** vulvovaginal warts, **b** HE ×20, **c** HE ×50, **d** HE ×100). FNA from left cervical lymph node revealed plenty of histiocytes containing large number of intracellular as well as extracellular capsulated organisms suggestive of *Histoplasma capsulatum* (**e** MGG ×400, **f** MGG ×1000, **g** HE ×400, **h** HE ×1000, **i** PAS ×400, and **j** PAS ×1000). Subsequently the patient developed ulceration in the left postauricular area and swab was obtained. The smear showed both intracellular and extracellular capsulated organisms suggestive of *Histoplasma* (*arrows*) along with plenty of Gram-positive cocci in clusters (**k**, **l** Giemsa ×1000). The aerobic culture showed the growth of *Staphylococcus aureus* which was methicillin sensitive. The patient was treated with antibiotics and itraconazole to which she responded (Contributors: Dr. Shalini Bhalla, Consultant Pathologist, and Dr Vipul Kumar Srivastava Consultant Microbiologist, Sahara Hospital, Lucknow, India)

Fig. 6.4 (continued)

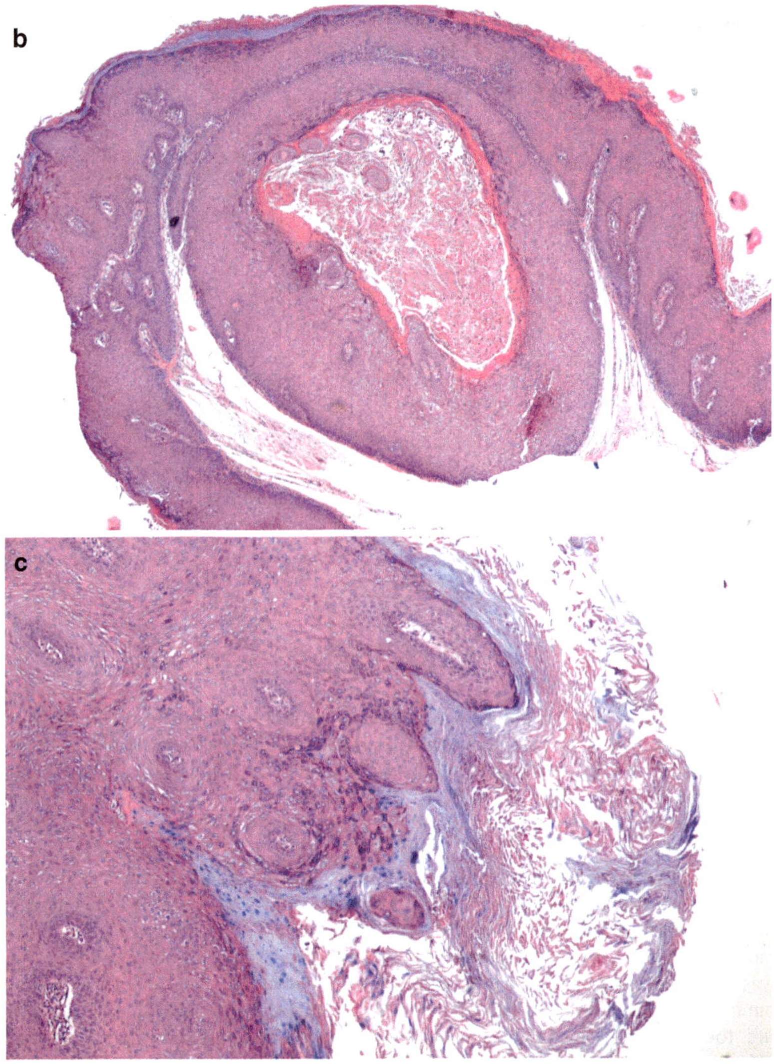

Fig. 6.4 (continued)

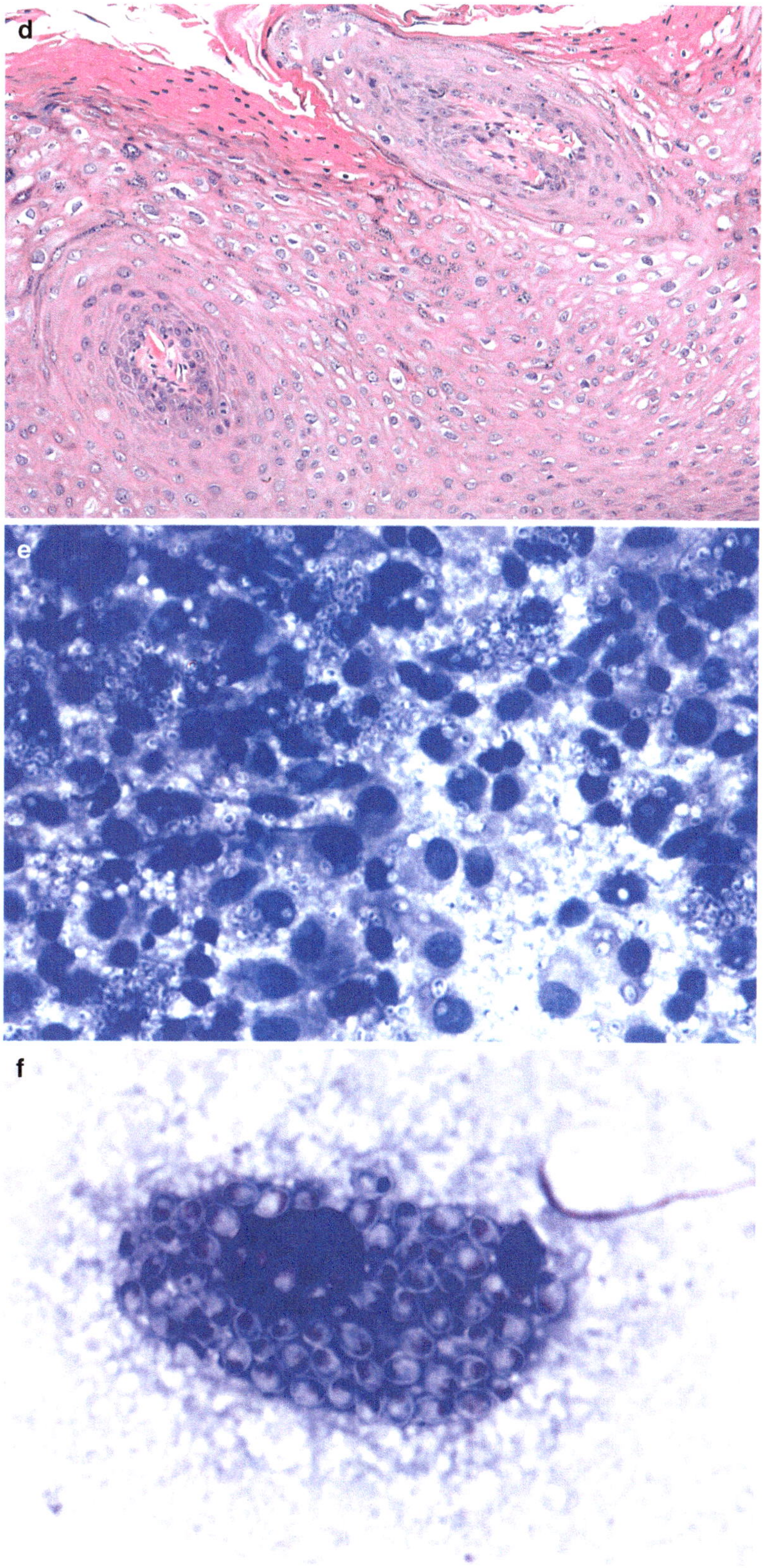

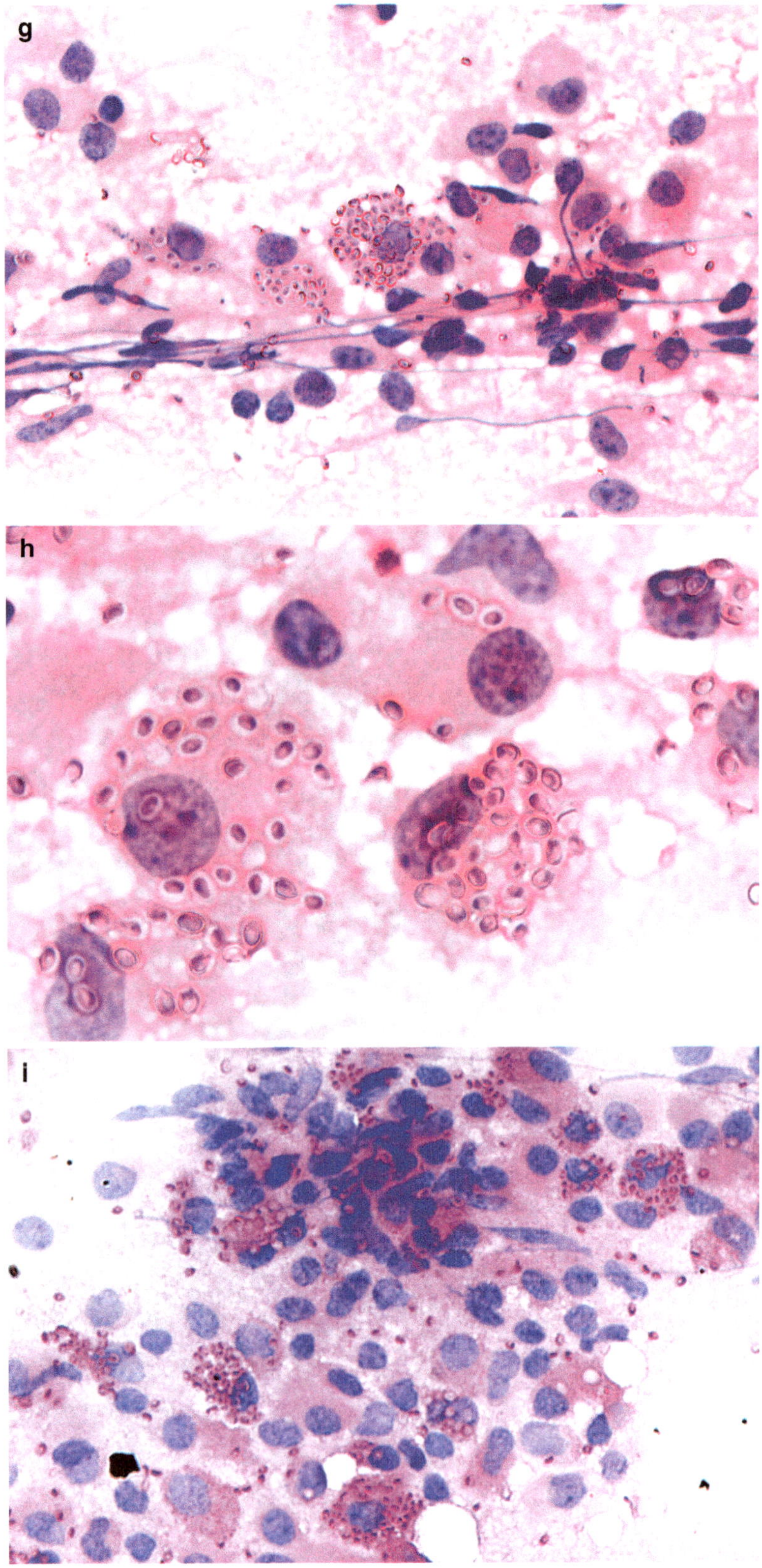

Fig. 6.4 (continued)

Fig. 6.4 (continued)

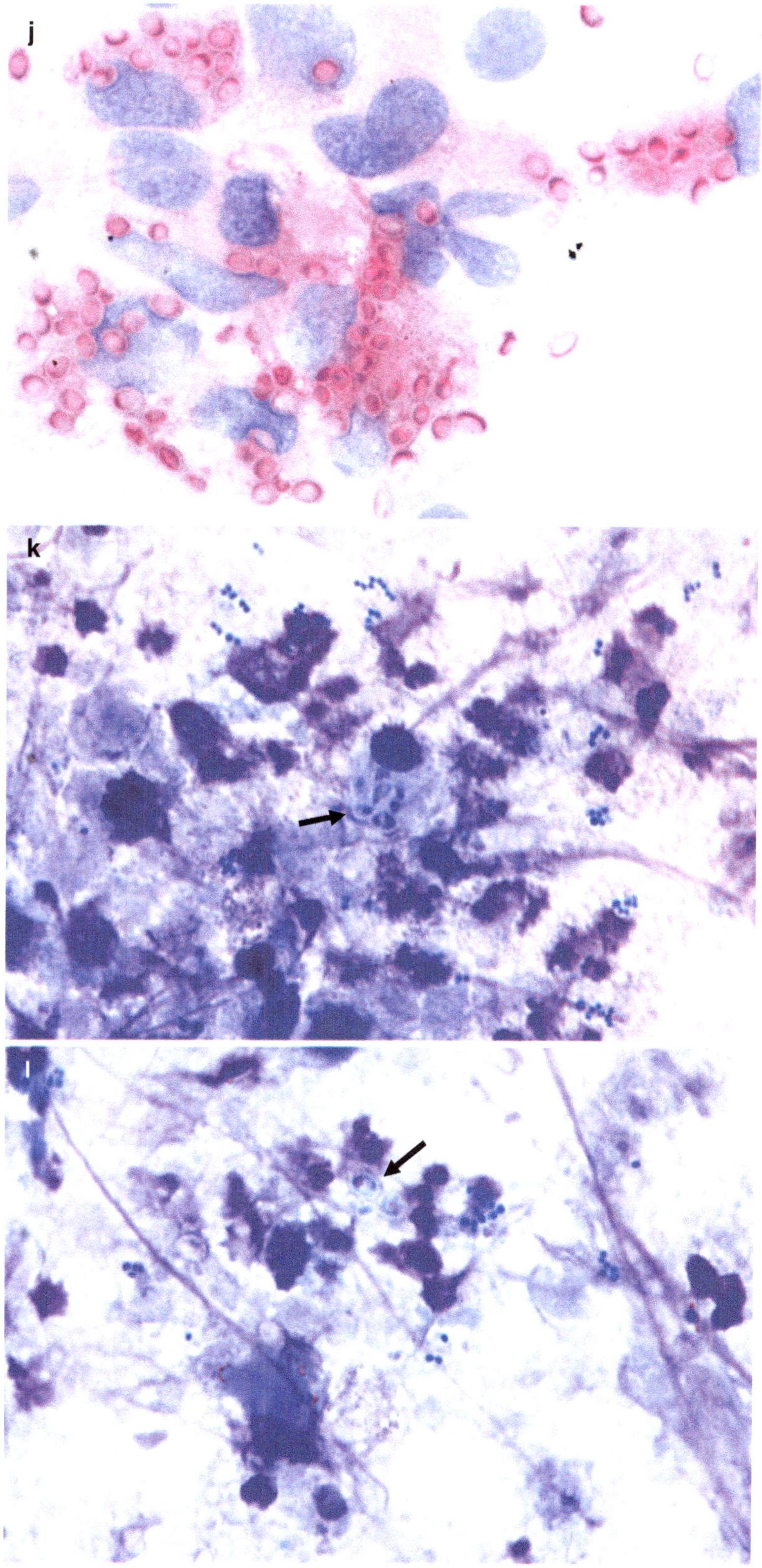

PTLD Stomach with CMV Disease in a Renal Allograft Recipient

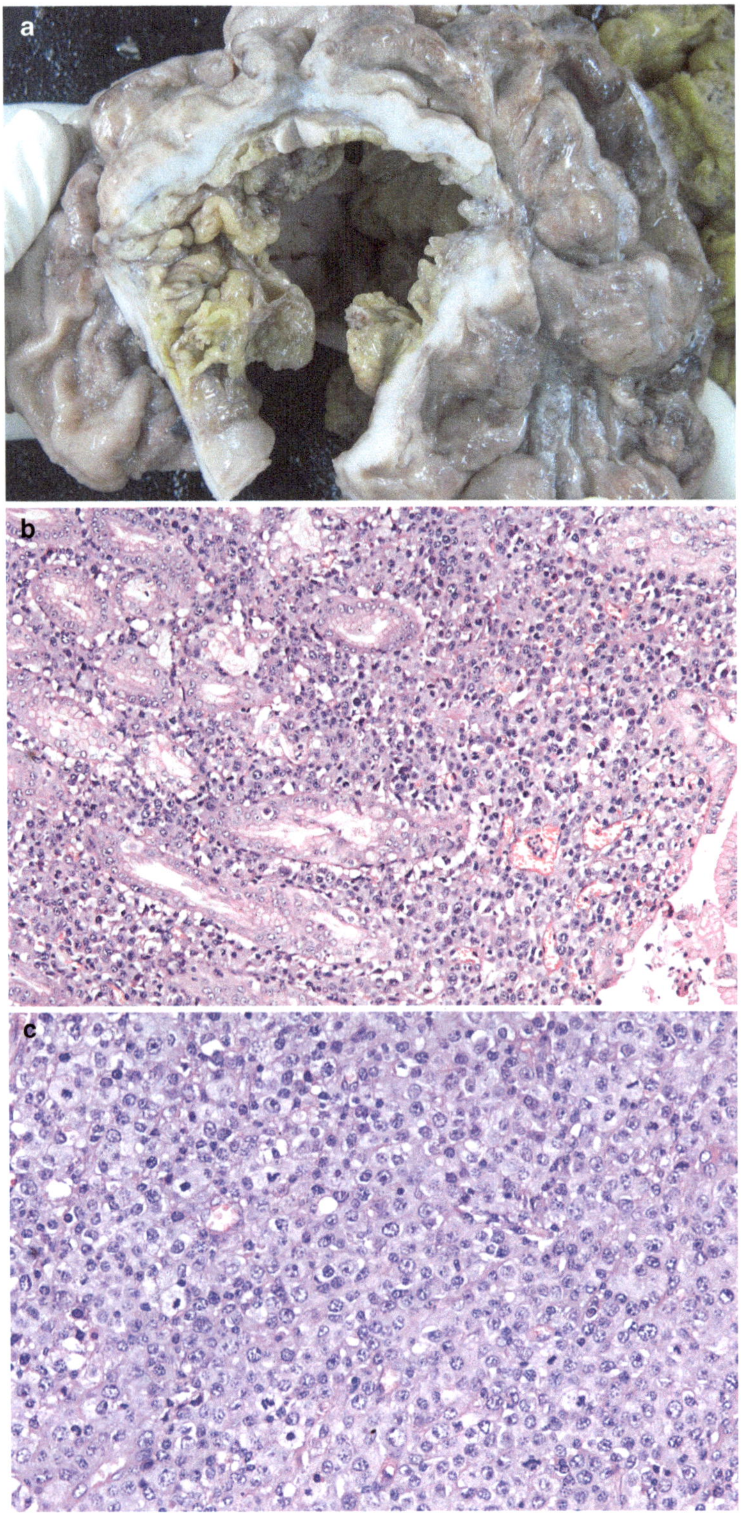

Fig. 6.5 (**a**–**j**) A 37-year-old male patient receiving live-related renal allograft for end-stage renal disease in the year 1999 was being maintained on triple drug immunosuppression. Four years later he developed pulmonary tuberculosis for which he received full course of ATT and deemed cured. Twelve years posttransplant, he presented with recurrent abdominal pain, loss of appetite, and occasional vomiting for the past 4 months. He was mildly anemic (Hb 9.5 g/dl); other laboratory parameters were WNL. Upper GI endoscopy revealed nodular swelling with sloughed mucosa in the antrum. Endoscopic biopsy revealed monomorphic diffuse large B-cell lymphoma (PTLD). Total gastrectomy was performed; besides the presence of monomorphic diffuse large B-cell lymphoma, the specimen also showed *H. pylori*-associated gastritis, and the gastric glands contained plenty of *H. pylori* (**a** gross specimen, **b** HE ×100, **c** HE ×200, **d**, **e** HE ×400, **f**–**i** IHC ×200). The gastric mucosa also showed cytomegaly and nucleomegaly with the presence of owl eye-like intranuclear inclusions suggestive of CMV gastritis (*arrow*) (**j** HE ×400). PCR for CMV was positive (Contributor – Prof. N Krishnani, Department of Pathology, Sanjay Gandhi Postgraduate Institute of Medical Sciences, Lucknow, India)

Fig. 6.5 (continued)

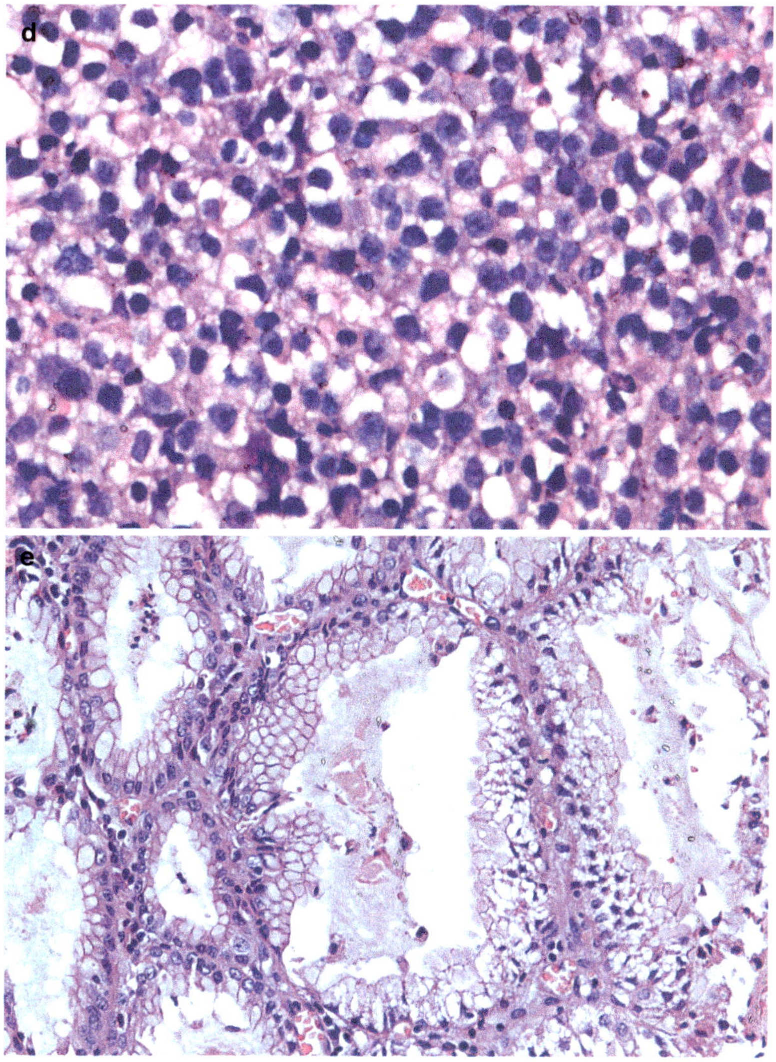

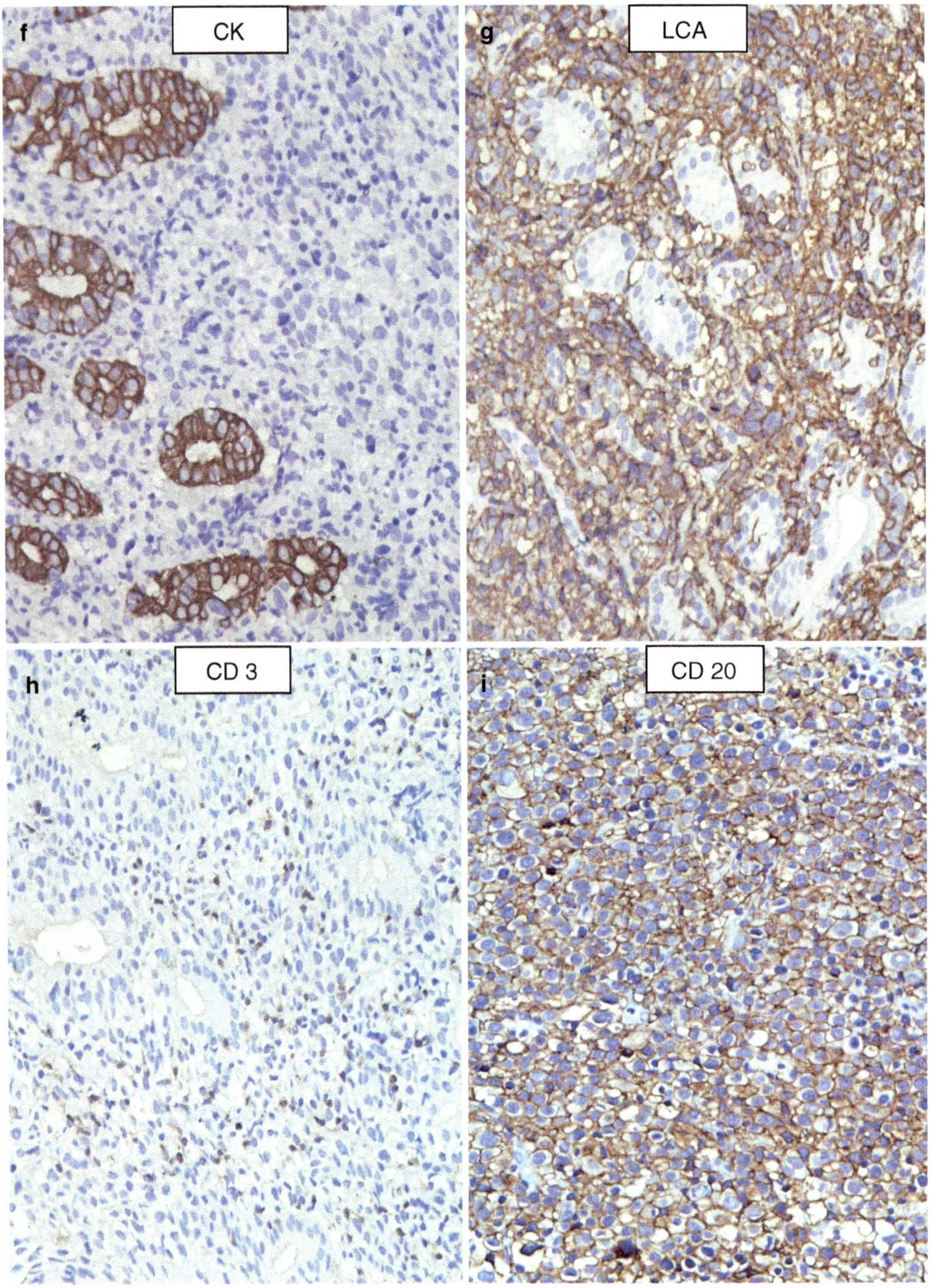

Fig. 6.5 (continued)

Fig. 6.5 (continued)

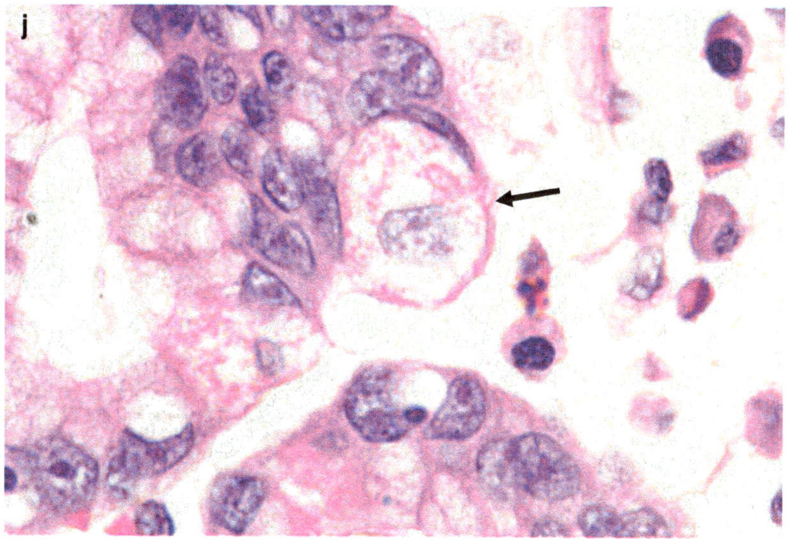

Zygomycosis Paranasal Sinuses with Subcutaneous Candidal Abscess in a Patient of ALL

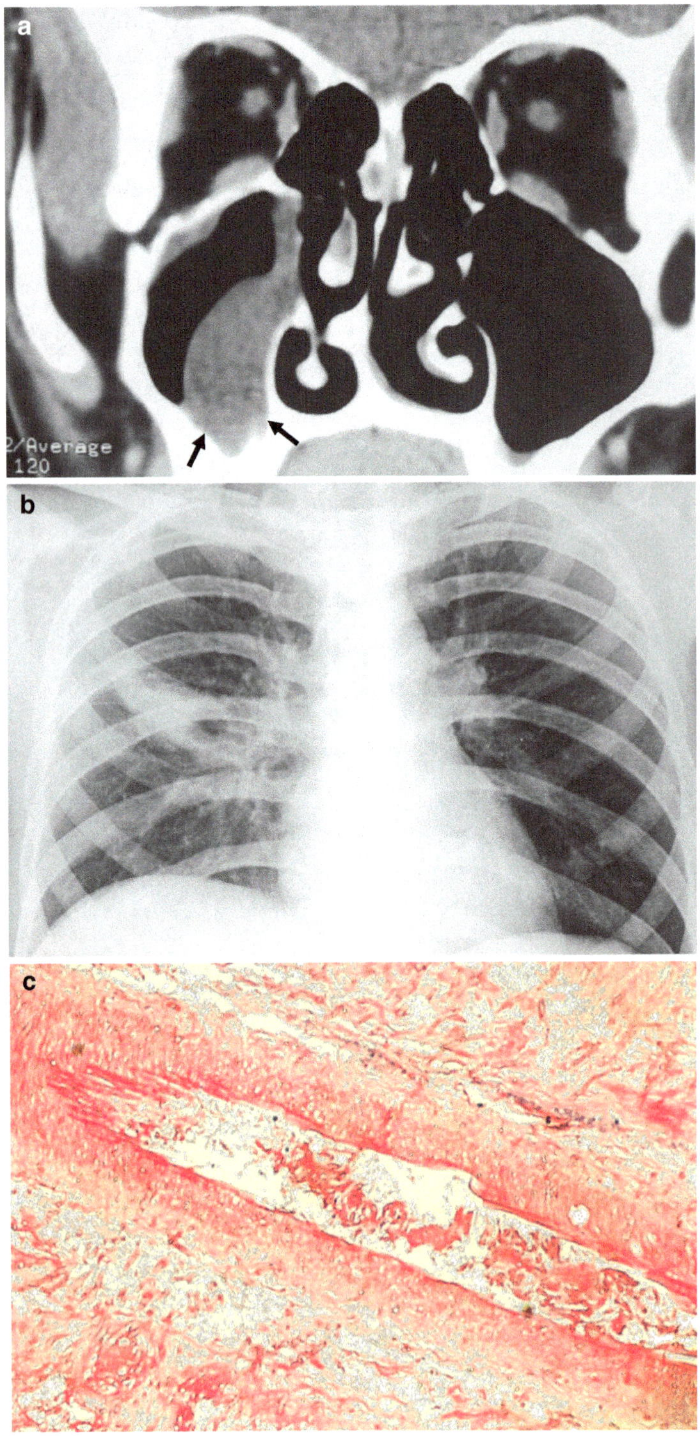

Fig. 6.6 (**a**–**g**) A 17-year-old male patient diagnosed as ALL (CALLA-positive B lineage) was undergoing treatment using BFM 90. ALL protocol received preinduction with corticosteroids. However, soon he was detected to have developed uncontrolled diabetes for which he received insulin as per sliding scale. He also received a dose of vincristine and two doses of L-asparaginase. At this time he was found to have pancytopenia. There after he developed bilateral nasal and palatal necrotizing mass lesions. CT showed mass in paranasal sinuses (**a**). Two weeks later patient developed a lesion in the right lung, and the X-ray chest showed it to be a cavitary lesion (**b**). Histological examination of the excised nasal mass revealed zygomycosis with angioinvasion. Subsequently the patient also developed multiple subcutaneous abscesses; the FNAC of the subcutaneous abscess showed yeasts and pseudo hyphae of *Candida* species as second fungal pathogen. Slide culture for fungus showed hyaline, branched, ribbon-shaped, aseptate hyphae with sporangiophores branching at the base with rhizoids. Sporangia are round with globose columella and pigmented spores characteristic of *Rhizopus* sp. (**c** HE ×400, **d** PAS ×400, **e** CSM ×400, and **f** lactophenol cotton blue ×400). Subsequently, while in the hospital, he also developed multiple subcutaneous abscesses; the FNAC showed yeasts and pseudo hyphae of *Candida* (**g** PAS ×400) (Contributor to mycological workup: Dr. Vipul Kumar Srivastava, Consultant Microbiologist, Sahara Hospital, Lucknow, India)

Fig. 6.6 (continued)

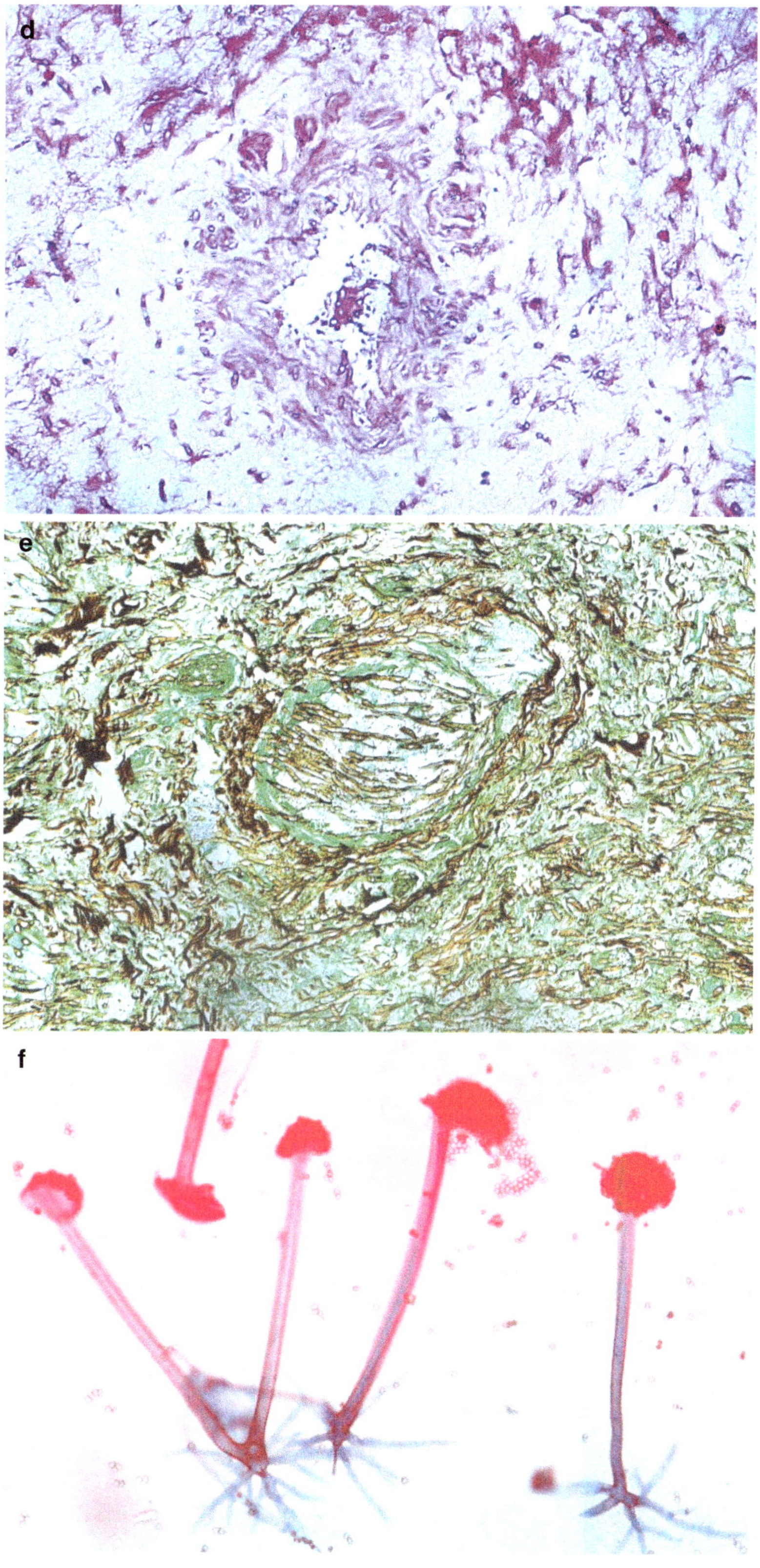

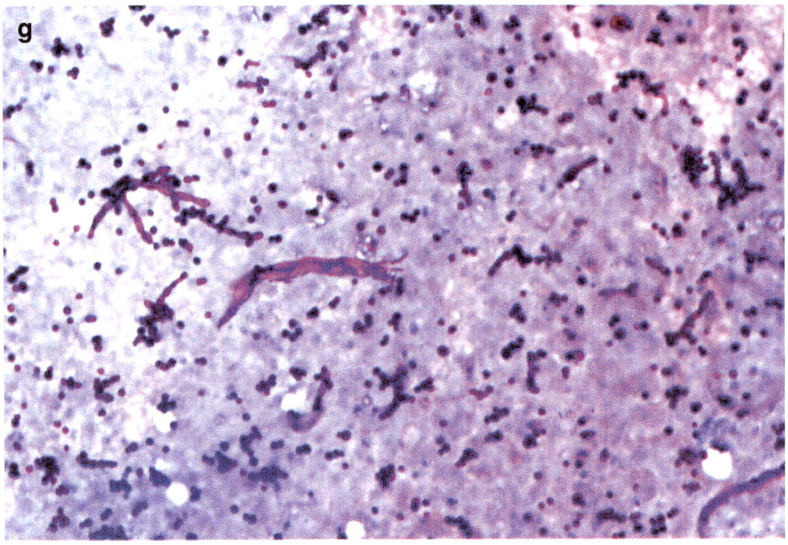

Fig. 6.6 (continued)

Zygomycosis with Candida in Oral Ulcer in a Patient of AML on Chemotherapy

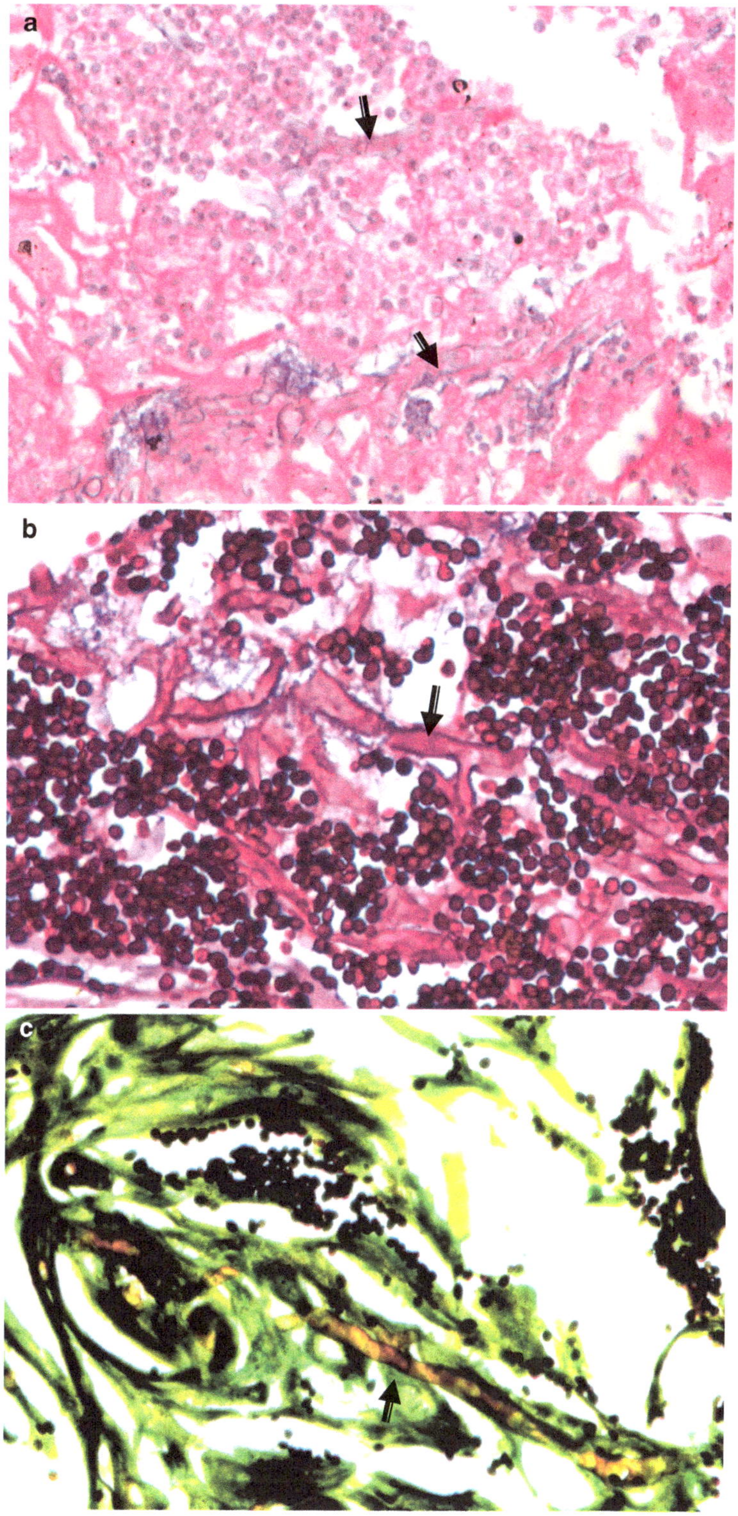

Fig. 6.7 (**a**–**c**) A 47-year-old female patient presented with pyrexia, progressively increasing weakness, and pallor for 20 days. She had no lymphadenopathy or hepatosplenomegaly. Laboratory workup revealed her to be suffering from acute myeloid leukemia – M2. She received induction therapy as per standard protocol. While in the hospital, she developed an ulcerated swelling in the left maxillary area; a biopsy from the lesion was obtained. Histological examination revealed plenty of budding yeastlike bodies with pseudo hyphae of *Candida* along with another filamentous fungus showing right angle branching aseptate hyaline hyphae having thick irregular walls suggestive of zygomycosis (*arrows*) as coexistent second fungal pathogen (**a** HE ×400, **b** PAS ×400, and **c** CSM ×400)

Candida with *Mucor* Involving the Soft Palate in a Debilitated Ill Patient

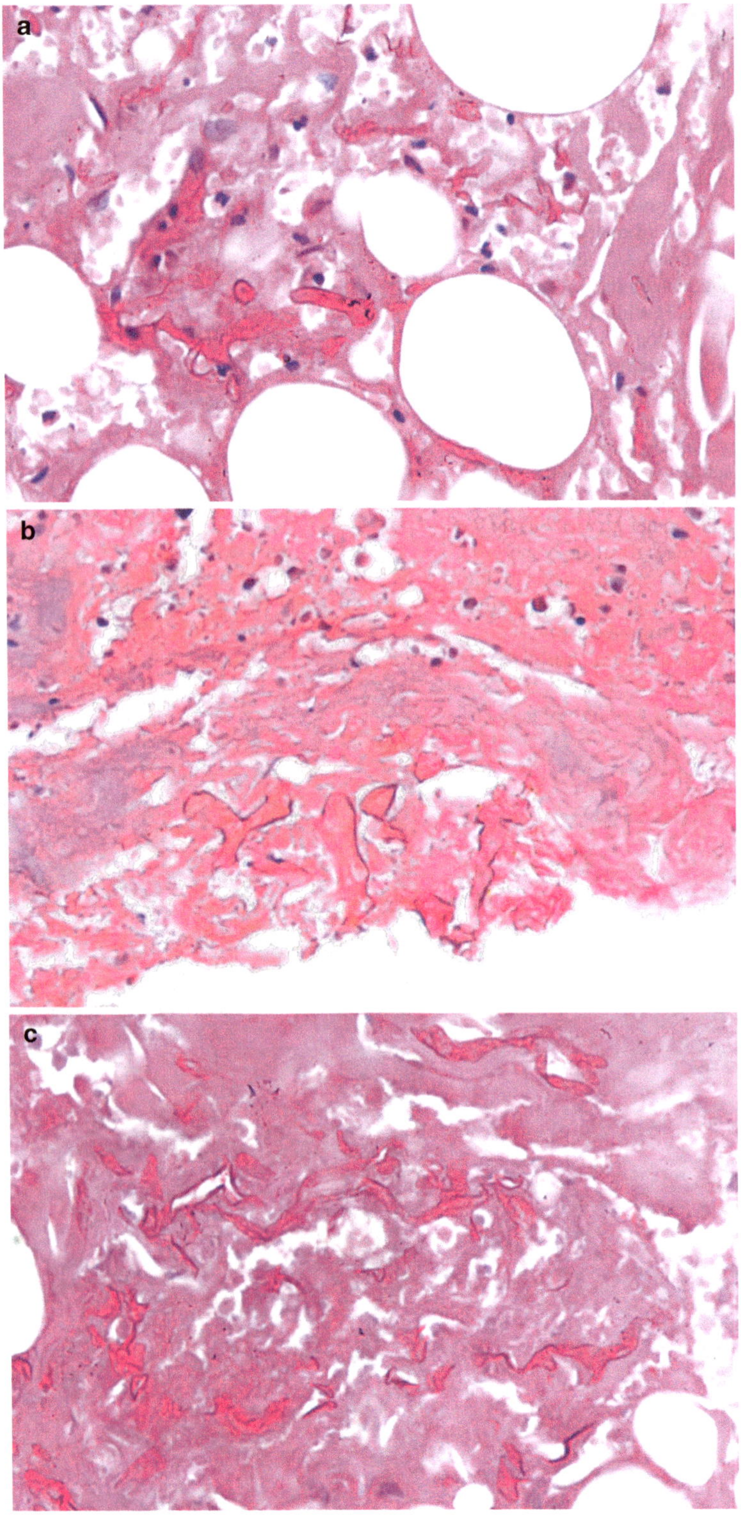

Fig. 6.8 (**a–d**) A 36-year-old female patient was admitted to the hospital with high-grade fever for 1 week with septicemia. Laboratory workup revealed hemoglobin content of 8.1 g/dl, total WBC count was 15,900/cu mm with 82 % polymorphs, and the platelets were 21,000/cu mm. Her blood urea was 103 mg/dl. Endotracheal aspirate showed the growth of *Acinetobacter*. During the course of hospital stay, she developed a blackish ulcerated swelling in the soft palate; a biopsy from the ulcerated area was obtained. Histological examination showed colonization with *Candida* (**a** PAS ×400) along with another fungus consisting of broad irregular aseptate thick-walled hyphae of *Mucor* showing tissue and angioinvasion (**b** HE ×400, **c** PAS ×400, and **d** CSM ×400)

Fig. 6.8 (continued)

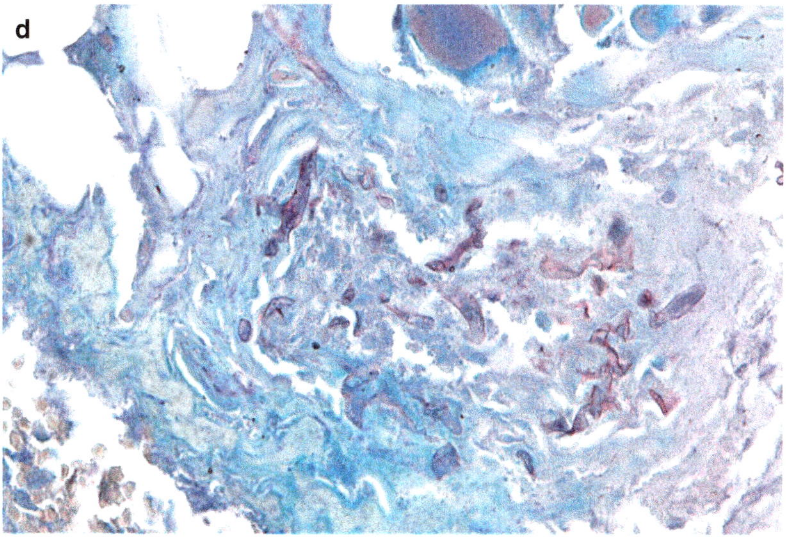

***Strongyloides* with *Giardia* Duodenum in an Immunocompromised Patient**

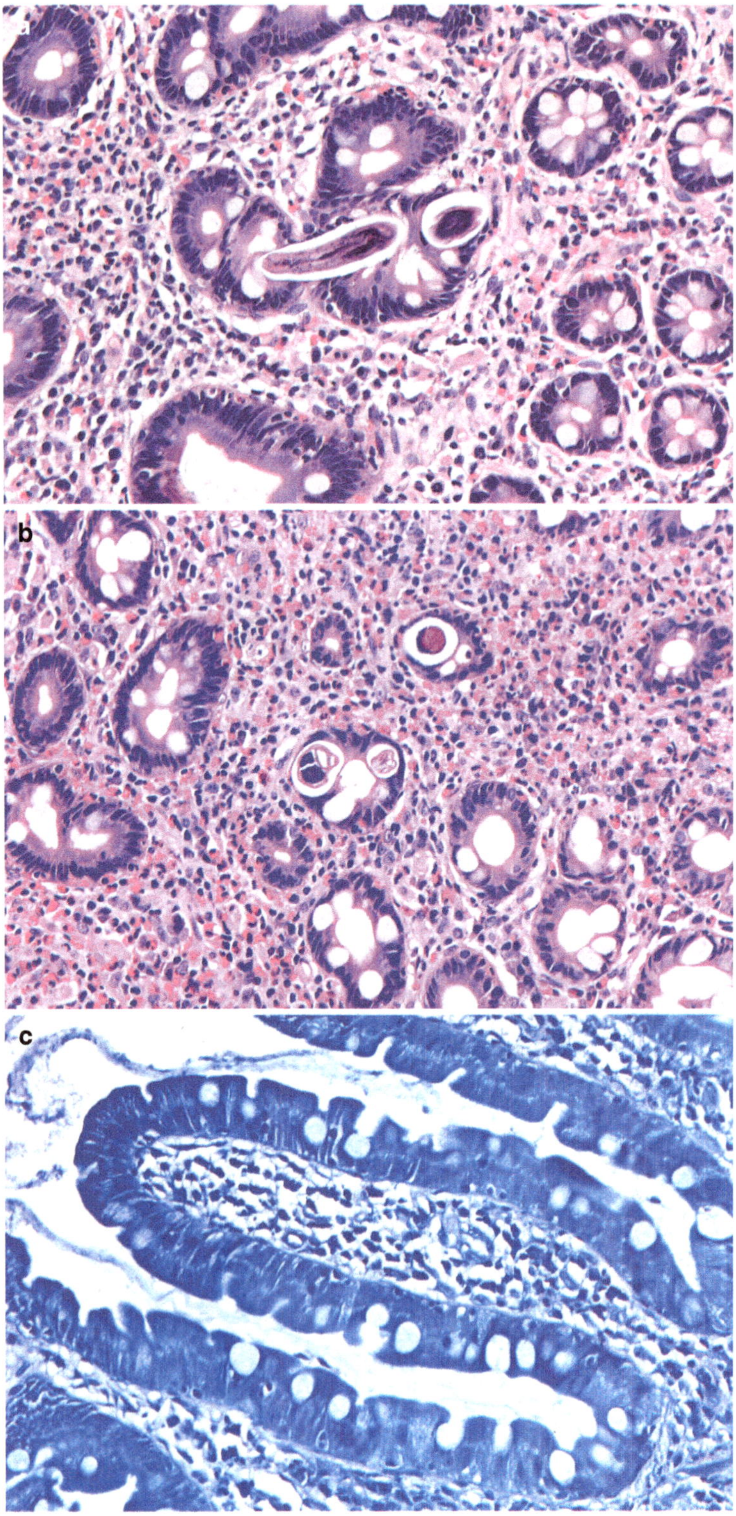

Fig. 6.9 (**a–c**) A 70-year-old female patient, a known case of osteoarthritis on prolonged steroid therapy, presented with upper abdominal pain for 1 month. Laboratory workup revealed TLC 22,200/cu mm with 52 % eosinophils. She was not diabetic. Other laboratory parameters were WNL. Serology for viral markers including HIV 1 and 2 was negative. CT abdomen revealed mild hepatomegaly, multiple enlarged mesenteric lymph nodes, and thickened DJ folds. Upper GI endoscopy revealed antral erosion as well as thickening and erosion of the mucosa of D1 and D2. Duodenal biopsy showed larvae of *Strongyloides* along with the presence of trophozoites of *Giardia* in duodenal crypts; the lamina showed dense eosinophilic infiltration (**a**, **b** HE ×200, **c** Giemsa ×200)

Appendix of Stains

Chromic Acid Silver Methenamine (CSM) Stain

Reagents

1. Chromic acid 5 %
2. Stock solution of 5 % silver nitrate 5 ml + 3 % hexamine (silver methenamine solution)
3. Borax solution 5 %
4. Sodium thiosulphate 3 %
5. Light green 0.2 %
6. Sodium or potassium metabisulphite 1 %

Working solution of silver methenamine is freshly prepared by mixing the following:

Stock solution of silver methenamine: 5 ml
5 % borax solution: 3 ml
Distilled water: 8 ml

Method

1. Section to water
2. Oxidize with 5 % chromic acid
3. Rinse in 1 % sodium or potassium metabisulphite
4. Wash in running water
5. Incubate in freshly prepared silver methenamine working solution at 58–60 °C for 30–60 min
6. Rinse in distilled water
7. Rinse with sodium thiosulphate
8. Wash in distilled water
9. Counter stain with light green.
10. Dehydrate, clear, and mount in DPX

Interpretation

Silver stain-positive organism – black
Background – pale green

Crystal Violet Stain

Reagents

Crystal violet solution:

- Dissolve 2 g crystal violet in 20 ml 95 % alcohol and add 80 ml 1 % ammonium oxalate.
- Dissolve using minimum of heat.

Method

1. Section to water.
2. Stain in crystal violet solution for 5 min.
3. Wash and differentiate in weak (0.2 %) acetic acid.
4. Wash and mount in glycerol.

Interpretation

Organisms – red purple
Background – blue

Giemsa Stain

Reagents

Giemsa stain

R.K. Gupta, P. Gupta (eds.), *Pathology of Opportunistic Infections*,
DOI 10.1007/978-981-10-1669-1

Method

1. Keep section in 2% Giemsa prepared in distilled water for 2 h.
2. Wash and mount.

Interpretation

Organisms – dark blue
Background – pale blue

Gram Stain

Reagents

1. Crystal violet solution – 0.5% crystal violet in 25% alcohol
2. Gram's and Lugo's iodine
   Iodine: 1 g
   Potassium iodide: 2 g
   Distilled water: 10 ml

   Shake and grind until dissolved. Make up to 300 ml with distilled water for Gram's iodine or 10 ml for Lugol's iodine.

3. 1% aqueous neutral red

Method

1. Section to water.
2. Stain with filtered crystal violet solution – 2 min.
3. Rinse with tap water.
4. Pour iodine solution – 2 min.
5. Wash with acetone.
6. Rinse in tap water.
7. Counterstain with neutral red for 3 min.
8. Blot, dehydrate, clear, and mount in DPX.

Interpretation

Gram-positive organisms – blue black
Gram-negative organisms – red

India Ink Preparation (for Cerebrospinal Fluid)

Reagent

India ink

Method

1. Centrifuge CSF.
2. Discard supernatant.
3. 1drop of sediment is mixed with 1 drop of India ink on a slide.
4. Cover with coverslip.

Interpretation

Cryptococci – negative shadow
Background – black

Kinyoun Stain (for Smears)

Reagents

1. Kinyoun's carbol fuchsin:
   Basic fuchsin: 4 g
   Phenol: 8 g
   Acid alcohol: 20 ml
   Distilled water: 100 ml
2. Sulphuric acid 1 %
3. Loeffler's alkaline methylene blue

   Dissolve 0.3 g of methylene blue in 30 ml of 95 % ethanol. Add 100 ml of 0.01 % potassium hydroxide.

Method

1. Prepare smear.
2. Allow to dry and fix by heat.
3. Flood slide with carbol fuchsin for 3 min.
4. Wash in running water.
5. Decolourize with 1 % H_2SO_4 for 10 s.
6. Wash in water.
7. Counterstain with methylene blue for 30 s.
8. Dry in air.

Interpretation

Acid-fast organisms – magenta
Background – blue

Masson's Fontana Stain

Reagents

Silver solution:

To a 20 ml of 10 % silver nitrate, concentrated NH_3 is added drop by drop until precipitate dissolves. When clear, add 20 ml of distilled water.

Method

1. Treat the section with silver solution; keep for 20 min at 60 °C in dark.
2. Wash with distilled water.
3. Treat with sodium thiosulphate.
4. Counterstain in 1 % neutral red.
5. Wash in water.
6. Dehydrate, clear, dry, and mount.

Interpretation

Organisms – black
Nuclei – red

Papanicolaou Stain

Reagents

1. Harris hematoxylin
2. OG 6 – orange G stock solution 100 ml (0.5 % in 95 % ethyl alcohol)
3. EA 50 (composition):
   - Light green SF (0.1 % in 95% alcohol): 45 ml
   - Bismark brown (0.5% in 95% alcohol): 10 ml
   - Eosin yellowish (0.5% in 95% alcohol): 45 ml
   - Phosphotungstic acid 0.2 g
   - Saturated lithium carbonate 1 drop

Method

1. Fix smears in 95 % alcohol.
2. Rinse slide in 95 % alcohol.
3. Rinse slide in 70 % alcohol.
4. Rinse slide in 95 % alcohol.
5. Rinse slide in distilled water.
6. Stain with Harris hematoxylin for 5–30 s.
7. Wash with distilled water.
8. Rinse in 1 % acid alcohol.
9. Rinse in 95 % alcohol.
10. Stain slide in OG 6 for 90 s.
11. Rinse slide in 95 % alcohol twice.
12. Stain slide EA 50 for 90 s.
13. Rinse slide in 95 % alcohol twice.
14. Rinse slide in absolute alcohol.
15. Dry and mount.

Interpretation

Organism – blue green
Nuclei – blue

Periodic Acid-Schiff (PAS) Stain

Reagents

1. Periodic acid Schiff 1 %
2. Schiff reagent:
   - Dissolve 1 g basic fuchsin in 200 ml of boiling distilled water and remove the flask from the heater.
   - Allow the solution to cool to 50 °C and add 2 g potassium metabisulphite with mixing.
   - Allow to cool to room temperature and then add 2 ml conc. HCl.
   - Mix and add 2 g activated charcoal and leave overnight in the dark at room temperature.
   - Filter through Whatman's no. 1 filter paper.
   - Store in a dark container at 4 °C

Method

1. Dewax and bring sections to water.
2. Treat with 1 % periodic acid Schiff – 5 min.
3. Wash well with several changes of distilled water.
4. Cover with Schiff solution – 30 min.
5. Wash in running water – 5 to 10 min.
6. Stain nuclei with Harris hematoxylin.
7. Differentiate as appropriate in 1 % acid alcohol and blue as usual.
8. Wash in water.
9. Dehydrate, clear, and mount in DPX.

Interpretation

PAS positive organisms – magenta
Nuclei – blue

Toluidine Blue Stain

Reagents

Toluidine blue solution:
1 % toluidine blue in 50 % isopropanol

Method

1. Section to water.
2. Cover with 1 % toluidine blue solution for 30 min at 37 °C.
3. Blot and place in absolute isopropanol for 1 min.
4. Clear and mount.

Interpretation

All components – deep blue

Ziehl-Neelsen Stain for Acid-Fast Bacilli

Reagents

Carbol fuchsin solution:

- 1 g basic fuchsin is dissolved in 10 ml of absolute alcohol and 100 ml of 5 % aqueous phenol is added. Mixed well and filtered.

Method

1. Section to water.
2. Stain in Coplin jar with filtered carbol fuchsin at 60 °C temperature for 30–60 min.
3. Wash in running tap water.
4. Differentiate in 1 % acid alcohol until the background staining is removed.
5. Wash in running tap water.
6. Counterstain nuclei with 1 % methylene blue for 1 min.
7. Dehydrate, clear, and mount in DPX.

Interpretation

Acid-fast organisms – magenta
Background – pale blue

Index

R.K. Gupta, P. Gupta (eds.), *Pathology of Opportunistic Infections*,
DOI 10.1007/978-981-10-1669-1

Printed by Printforce, the Netherlands